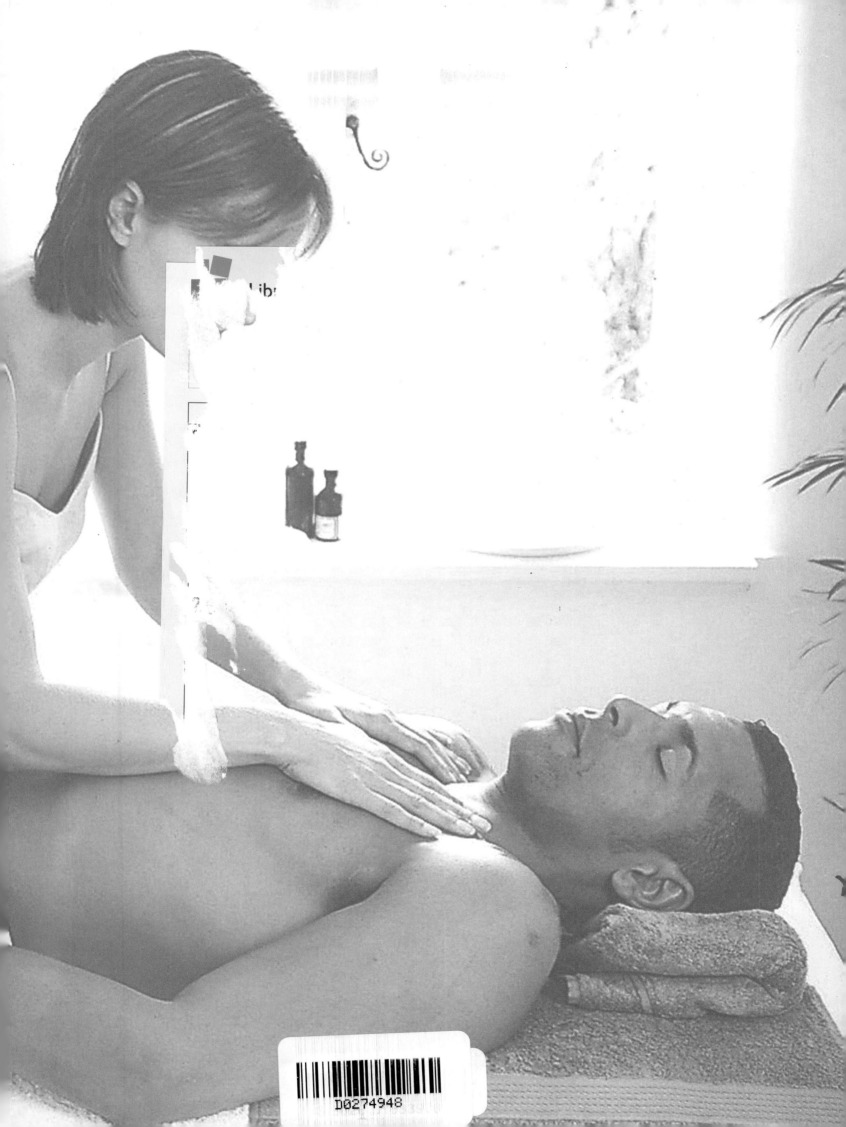

mind-blowing

HEAD MASSAGE

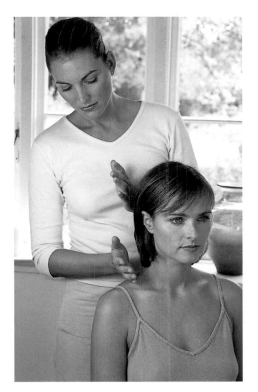

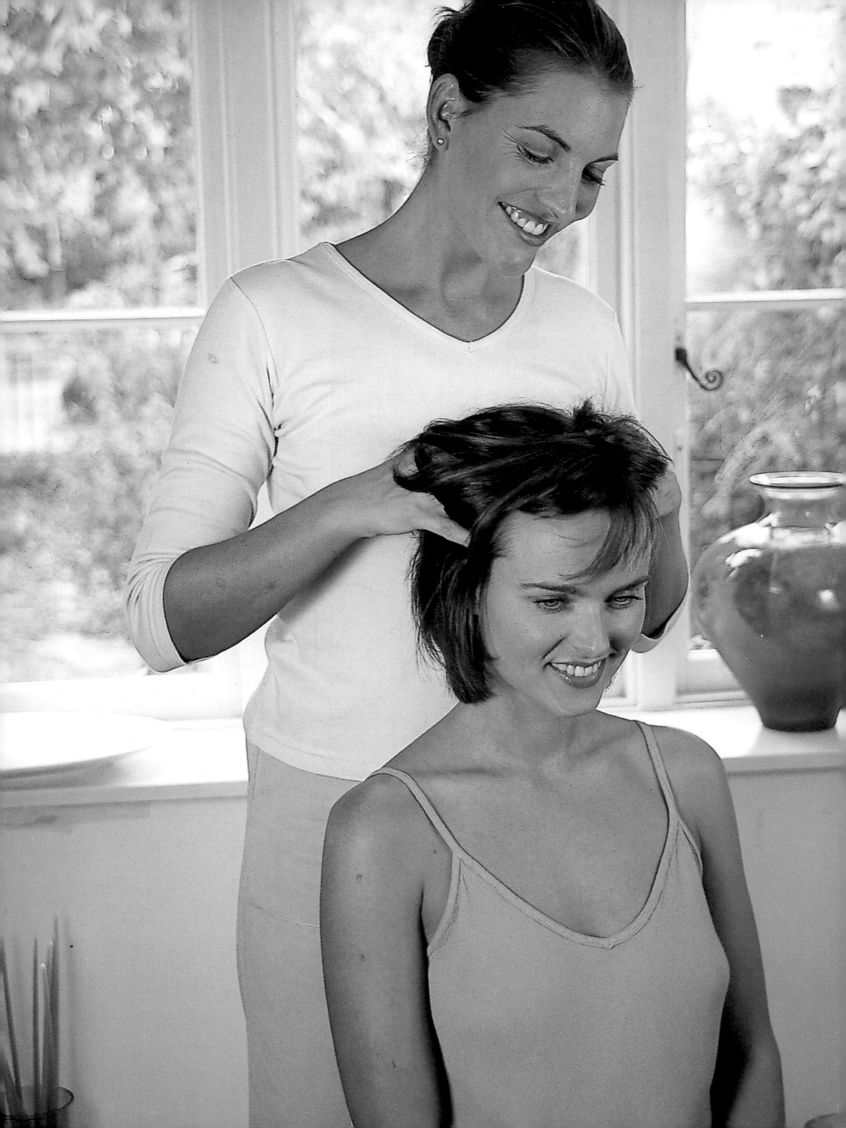

mind-blowing
HEAD MASSAGE

Traditional techniques of an ancient Indian
system revealed in step-by-step detail

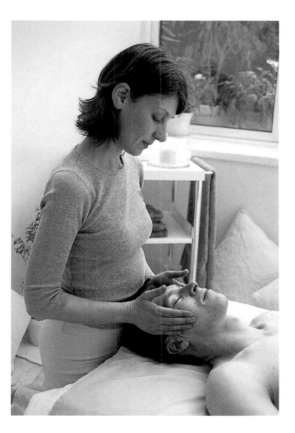

Francesca Rinaldi
photography by Michelle Garrett

LORENZ BOOKS

This edition is published by Lorenz Books

Lorenz Books is an imprint of Anness Publishing Ltd
Hermes House, 88–89 Blackfriars Road, London SE1 8HA
tel. 020 7401 2077; fax 020 7633 9499
www.lorenzbooks.com
info@anness.com

© Anness Publishing Ltd 2003

UK agent: The Manning Partnership Ltd, 6 The Old Dairy, Melcombe
Road, Bath BA2 3LR; tel. 01225 478444; fax 01225 478440;
sales@manning-partnership.co.uk

UK distributor: Grantham Book Services Ltd, Isaac Newton Way, Alma
Park Industrial Estate, Grantham, Lincs NG31 9SD; tel. 01476 541080;
fax 01476 541061; orders@gbs.tbs-ltd.co.uk

North American agent/distributor: National Book Network, 4501
Forbes Boulevard, Suite 200, Lanham, MD 20706; tel. 301 459 3366;
fax 301 429 5746; www.nbnbooks.com

Australian agent/distributor: Pan Macmillan Australia, Level 18, St
Martins Tower, 31 Market St, Sydney, NSW 2000; tel. 1300 135 113; fax
1300 135 103; customer.service@macmillan.com.au

New Zealand agent/distributor: David Bateman Ltd, 30 Tarndale
Grove, Off Bush Road, Albany, Auckland; tel. (09) 415 7664; fax (09)
415 8892

A CIP catalogue record for this book is available from the
British Library.

Publisher: Joanna Lorenz
Managing Editor: Helen Sudell
Senior Editor: Joanne Rippin
Designer: Nigel Partridge
Photographer: Michelle Garrett
Editorial Reader: Kate Humby
Production Controller: Darren Price

This book is not intended to replace advice from a qualified medical
practitioner. Please seek a medical opinion if you have any concerns
about your health. Neither the authors nor the publishers can accept
any liability for failure to follow this advice.

10 9 8 7 6 5 4 3 2 1

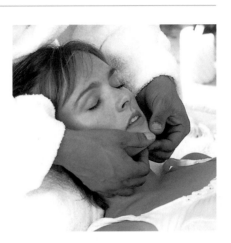
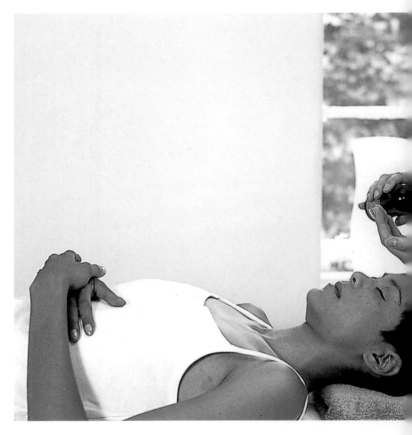
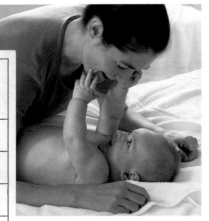

Contents

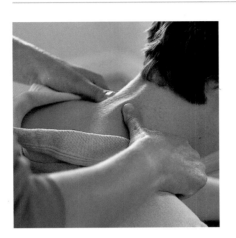

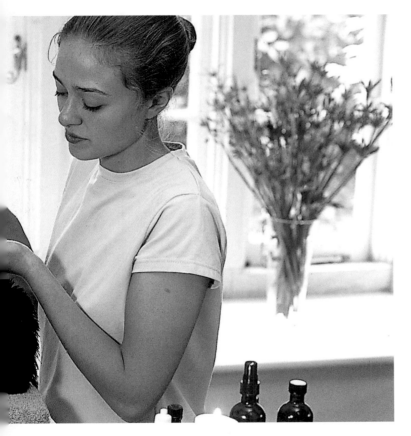

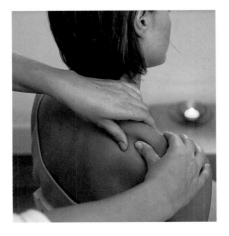

Introduction

Massage has seen an explosion of interest in recent years. This touch therapy is not only wonderful to receive, but it also has countless benefits. A massage treatment can relieve tension in the body, calm the mind, and nourish the soul, bringing healing on many different levels simultaneously. There is not just one type of massage however, but many different schools, each with its own style and approach. Indian head massage is just one of these.

approaches to massage

Broadly speaking there are two main approaches within massage: those that are "energy" based, and those that are more concerned with muscular physiology, though the trend is towards increasing integration. Energy-based approaches are influenced by ideas from the East, where it is widely believed that a universal life force enters and leaves the body at energy centres known as "chakras" and runs through the body along special channels, or "meridians". If this vital flow is blocked through tension or injury, then pain or illness will result. Energy-based techniques make use of thumb or finger pressure at the relevant points along the meridians to help release these energy blocks, enabling it to balance and flow freely once more through the body. They also focus on realigning the body's subtle energies through the chakra system.

In the West, we come from a tradition of muscular-based massage. This approach is more concerned with physiology and focuses on the muscular skeletal system. It is generally a fairly firm style of massage, and sports massage has grown out of this tradition. More recently, a growing trend has been the use of aromatic plant oils that are applied in massage for specific therapeutic effects. Known as "aromatherapy", this is a lighter style of massage and is concerned primarily with introducing the oils into the body through the medium of the skin. This type of massage is popular for its "feel-good" factor, as well as being particularly effective in treating problems that include a powerful emotional or mental component.

Indian head massage

With its origins in India, head massage is a relatively new addition to the different types of massage therapy available in the West, yet it is a newcomer that has caught on with great speed and popularity – perhaps because it captures the spirit of the modern age so well.

For centuries, head massage has played an essential part in Ayurvedic medicine, widely practised throughout India and parts of Asia. In India it is also a regular aspect of daily life. Travelling through India today, it is not unusual to see head massage practised on a street corner. However, this ancient art is highly practical and relevant to the Western world. Head massage is quick to receive, and does not involve stripping off or necessarily using oils. It is mess free, convenient and possible to do almost anywhere. It combines energy-based pressure-point techniques with more traditional massage strokes such as rubbing and stroking, thus working on the body's energy system as well as its physical structure. In addition to focusing on the head, it also targets the upper back, shoulders, and neck area – the significant places in the body where we store tension.

Head massage is also highly effective in dealing with a range of physical and emotional complaints, especially those that are stress related, while it can also form an essential part of pampering and body-care routines. What is more, head massage is easy to learn and can be done by almost anyone.

about this book

This book begins with an overview of the history of massage, before looking specifically at Indian head massage. It goes on to explain how traditional head massage can be adapted to suit a contemporary Western setting, where it can be enjoyed with friends as part of a pampering session or made part of your everyday health and beauty regime. It shows how head massage can be used to treat the symptoms of stress – both at home and at work – or to alleviate common conditions such as asthma, anxiety, headaches and sore sinuses, as well as body tension from driving or computer work. Information on using massage with babies and children is also included, as is a special section at the end that shows how to use different types of massage oils in pampering and beauty treatments for the hair and body.

Clear information is given on the basic massage strokes, and by following the step-by-step instructions you are guided through a head massage routine with a partner. This sequence is broken down into bite-size chunks, each one focusing on a different area, such as the upper back, shoulders and arms, and head to make it easy to learn and remember. Step sequences are also included for a self-massage routine, as well as shorter, quick-fix, stress-busting treatments to be used throughout the day.

What is contained here makes head massage accessible and easy to integrate into your everyday life, and the benefits of head massage are multifaceted. By working on the body with sensitivity and awareness, changes can be affected through the body's systems, encouraging relaxation and peace of mind, and bringing people back to themselves by harmonizing body and soul. It is also an immensely enjoyable way of spending time with friends and family.

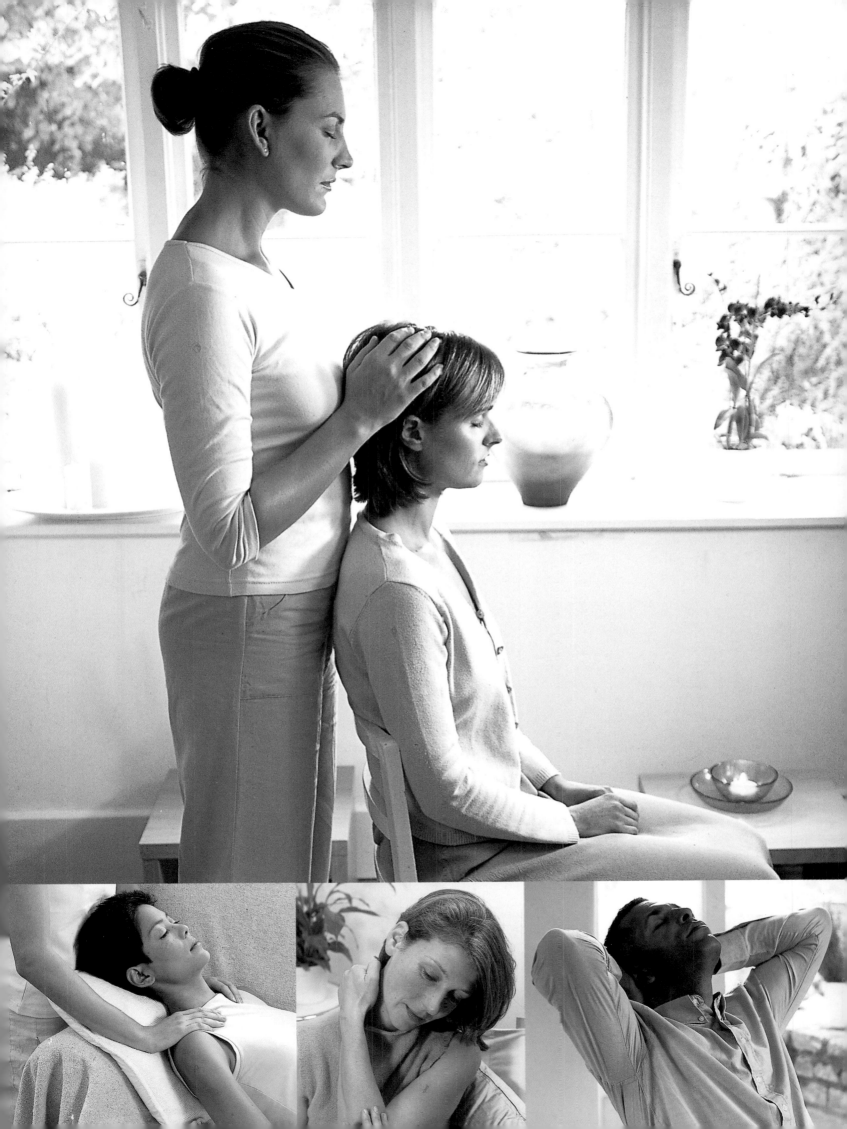

An Introduction to Massage

Massage is one of the oldest therapies in the world, with head massage being part of this age-old healing tradition. Based on therapeutic touch, massage speaks in a timeless and universal language that can be used to communicate warmth, give reassurance or alleviate aches and pains by sending healing signals to the brain. Today we are rediscovering this ancient art and adapting it to suit the needs of a modern lifestyle.

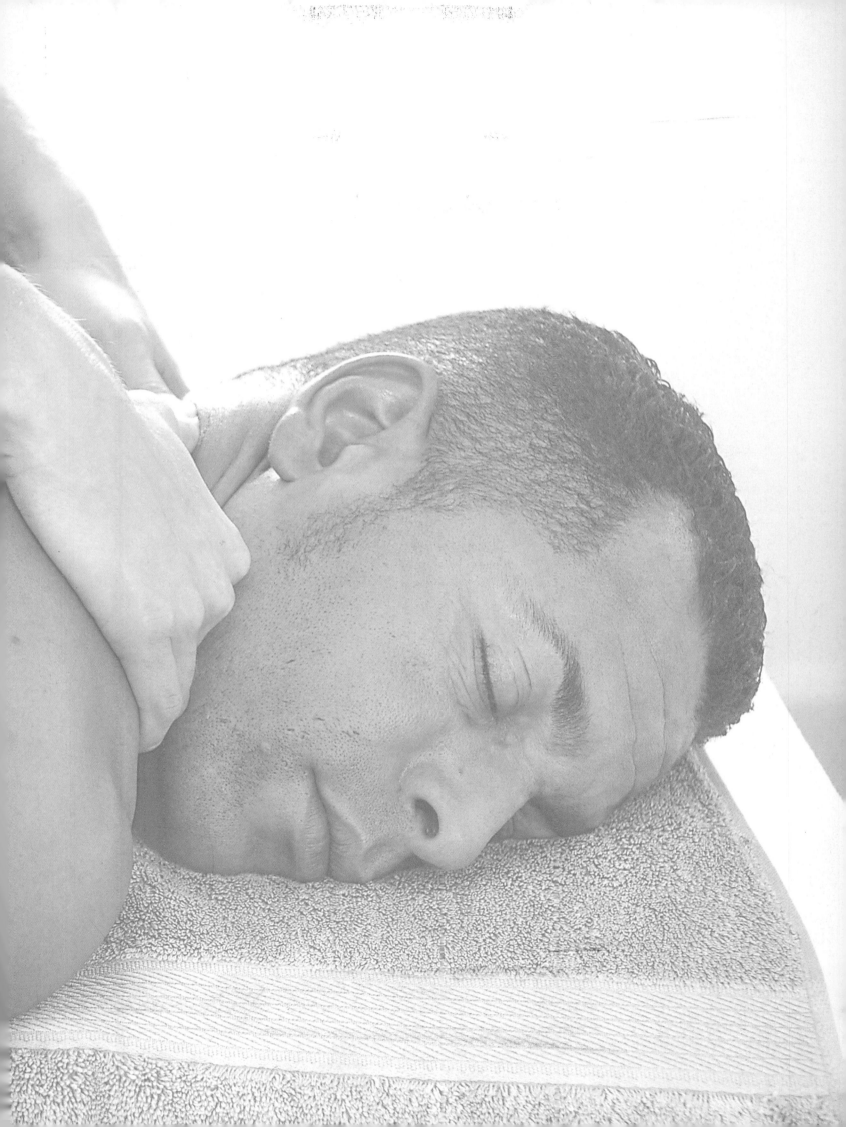

Massage in history

Massage is one of the oldest therapies in the world, yet to discover its precise origins is almost impossible. The use of touch for grooming, stroking and rubbing is a behaviour that we share with many animals. Touch is instinctive, and from here it is a small step to develop this natural ability into a healing art. There is evidence that every culture throughout the world has used massage in some form or other, and every language, ancient or modern, has a word for massage. In the East the tradition of massage has always been unbroken, although its practice has been more staggered and erratic in Western cultures.

the ancient and classical world

Ancient Chinese medical texts, dating back some 5000 years, advocate stroking the body to "protect against colds, keep the organs supple and prevent minor ailments".

Another text contains information that is akin to the passive limb movements used in modern Swedish massage. In India, Ayurvedic scripts from around 4000 years ago also recommend rubbing the body to treat and prevent disease. Since then massage has been inextricably linked with Indian culture. For instance, it is customary for a bride and groom to receive a massage before their wedding day, and most Indian mothers are taught how to massage their newborn babies and young children.

In ancient Egypt, *bas-relief* carvings dating back more than 4000 years show Pharaoh Ptah-Hotep receiving a leg massage from a male servant, while centuries later, Queen Cleopatra is recorded as enjoying a foot

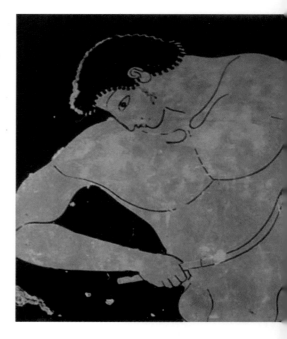

△ The Greeks used oil to cleanse themselves before bathing and massage. Here an athlete in a gymnasium removes the oil from his body.

▽ The Karma Sutra and ancient Ayurvedic scripts contain many references to sensual massage, which was used for pleasure, spiritual practice and general health and wellbeing.

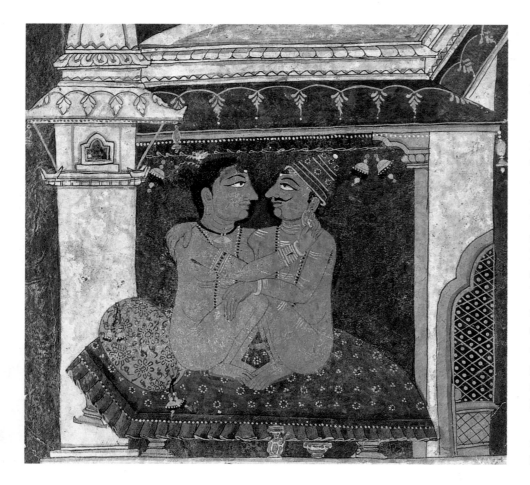

massage during dinner parties. However, enjoyment of massage was not restricted to the wealthy. Ancient records show that even the lowliest Egyptian workers were paid in wages of body oil sufficient for daily use.

For the ancient Greeks, the pursuit of physical excellence was paramount, and massage played an intrinsic part in their exaltation of the body. Their famous medical centres, or gymnasia, contained open-air training rooms, sports grounds and massage rooms. In ancient Greece, massage was highly recommended for treating fatigue, sports or war injuries, as well as illness. Writing in the 5th century BC, Hippocrates, the reputed "father of modern medicine", stated that a succesful physician must be experienced in the art of "rubbing", and prescribed a scented bath followed by a daily massage with oils as the pathway to good health and fitness.

The Romans were equally fond of massage and incorporated it into their bathing rituals. For the wealthy, it was

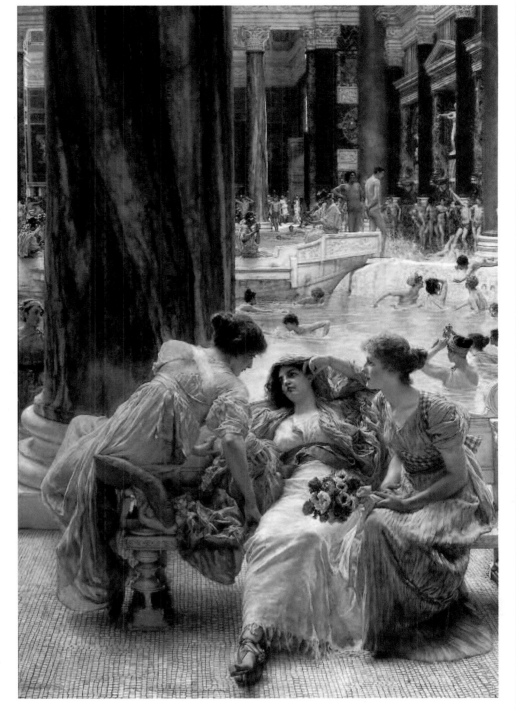

▷ **The Roman Empire saw a renaissance in interest in bodily pleasures and rituals, including massage and cleansing, which were practised in the ubiquitous Roman baths.**

customary to attend the baths and have stiff muscles rubbed with warm vegetable oil. This was followed by a full body massage to awaken the nerves, get the circulation going and mobilize the joints. The routine was completed as fine oil was liberally applied all over the body to nourish the skin and keep it fine and smooth. Physicians also promoted the therapeutic benefits of massage. One of the most famous of these was Galen (AD 130–201), who wrote books on massage, exercise and health. He also classified different massage strokes, and used massage in the treatment of many diseases.

the Middle Ages and beyond

After the decline of the Roman Empire, the Arab world became the centre of learning and culture. The works of Hippocrates, Galen and other famous physicians were translated into Arabic, preserving the medical knowledge built up since antiquity. Avicenna (980–1037), one of the greatest Arab physicians, added to this knowledge and went on to describe the use of healing plants, spinal manipulation and various forms of massage in great detail.

Meanwhile, in Europe, touch became associated with "carnal pleasures" in the eyes of the Catholic Church and massage was denounced as a highly sinful activity. Its practice was consigned to the realm of folklore, and knowledge was passed down through the female line – the local "wise woman" or midwife – along with knowledge of herbs and other healing remedies. This information was regarded with suspicion and could lead to persecution as a witch.

The Renaissance saw a revival of interest in classical medicine, and massage gradually became more respected by mainstream society. Ambroise Paré, a 16th-century physician to the French court, used massage in his practice. European journeys of exploration also revealed how other cultures valued massage. Captain Cook described

how massage cured his sciatic pains in Tahiti, and in the 1800s there are records of the Cherokee and Navaho Indians using massage treatments on their warriors.

towards the modern age

However it was at the end of the 19th century that a Swedish gymnast, Per Henrik Ling (1776–1839), restored to favour therapeutic massage in Europe. Having cured himself of rheumatism, Ling developed a system of massage that was based on physiology, gymnastic movements and massage. Receiving royal patronage for his work, Ling's methods laid the foundation for modern physiotherapy with the

establishment in 1894 of the Society of Trained Masseurs. A few years later, St George's Hospital in London opened a massage department, and "Swedish" massage therapy soon became part of mainstream medical practice.

This emphasis continued unchecked until the 1960s, when personal growth centres, notably the Esalen Institute in California, adapted massage therapy into a holistic treatment that could balance mind, body and emotions, rather than simply relieving muscular aches and pains. This holistic approach is now widely used alongside mainstream medicine as a complement to conventional medical treatments.

Indian head massage

Unlike many other healing traditions, Indian head massage is as widely practised today as it was thousands of years ago. It has its roots in Ayurveda, one of the oldest healthcare systems in the world. Dating back more than 4000 years, Ayurveda is grounded in the philosophical and spiritual traditions of India. It offers comprehensive and practical guidelines for how to achieve health and wellbeing, and covers many different aspects of daily life.

the science of longevity

Ayurveda is known as the "science of longevity". It is based upon the holistic principle that illness or disease is created when we are out of balance. It describes three energy forces (known as the *doshas*) namely *vata*, *pitta* and *kapha*, each having its own characteristics and purpose. All physical, emotional and mental functions are controlled by the *doshas*. When they are balanced and working in harmony, we feel vibrant and enjoy good health.

▽ **Indian women have been admired throughout history for their long, lustrous, thick black hair that is traditionally nourished, maintained and groomed with oils and by head massage.**

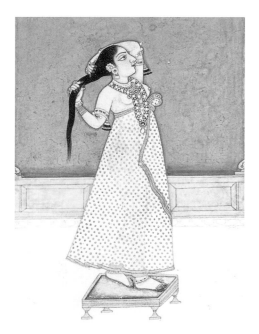

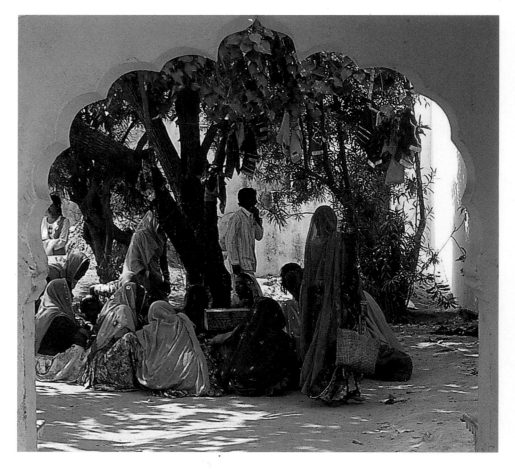

The Ayurvedic healthcare regime is comprehensive. It covers diet and exercise, yoga and meditation, detox and herbal remedies, as well as regular massage treatments using essential oils. A weekly head massage is highly recommended as a way of restoring and maintaining balance in the body's systems. Specific oils and herbs are used with head massage to help to stabilize the *doshas*. For instance, a *vata*-type imbalance may manifest as dry skin and hair, in which case sesame oil, with its strengthening and nourishing properties, would be recommended.

touch culture

The healing power of touch to restore and maintain wellbeing is deeply embedded in the culture of India, and head massage has to be seen within this context. Massage plays an important part in many major life events, such as marriage and pregnancy, or

△ **An Indian wedding is about to begin. The ritual of preparing the bride and groom for the ceremony will have included head massage.**

in looking after babies and children. It is customary to give massage to both the bride and groom before they get married. This involves ritual and the use of specially blended herbs and oils designed to strengthen, beautify and bless the couple in preparation for marriage.

The practice of baby massage is also widespread. Even at the poorest level of society, where people live on the streets, and deprivation and hunger are rife, mothers can be seen oiling and massaging their babies every day, regardless of the traffic, dogs, pedestrians and street sellers all around them. In India, massage is not seen as a luxury, but as one of life's essentials. Daily massage continues until the child is about three years old, when it is reduced to twice a week. From the age of six, children then take part in a weekly massage ritual with other members of the family, even learning to exchange massage with one another.

male and female traditions

Historically the practice of Indian head massage is carried through both the female and male line, each having a different emphasis. The female line is primarily concerned with grooming, bonding and nurturing. Every week, head massage is carried out in the family home, where mothers nourish and condition their children's hair with oils and scalp rubs. For daughters and women, the weekly ritual is elaborate and time-consuming, involving lengthy preparations. That is because in India a woman's hair carries great status, so taking

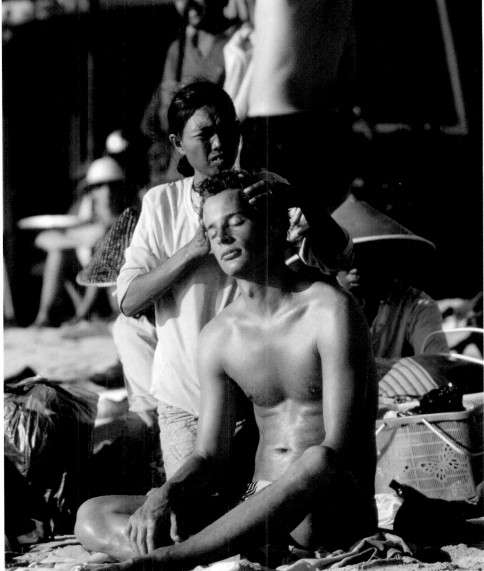

△ In India head massage is traditionally practised on the streets by male masseurs. In areas frequented by tourists, however, women have taken up this public work.

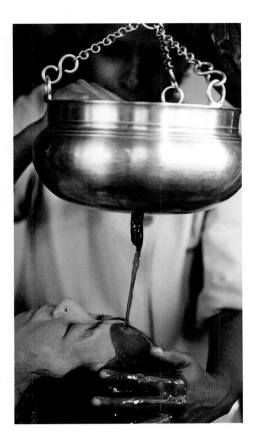

▽ *Shirodhara*, the sensual ritual of running warmed sesame oil on to the middle of the forehead, is a relaxing and therapeutic part of traditional Ayurvedic practice.

care of it is extremely important. There are many different traditions and ways of doing this. In the villages, it is usually a communal outdoor activity. Women of all ages get together once a week and sit in the sunshine to indulge in head massage and brush and groom each other's hair. The heat of the sun allows the oils to penetrate into the hair shaft, nourishing and conditioning it. The ritual is very much a social activity that gives the women involved a chance to talk and relax with one another.

Men also enjoy a tradition of head massage, which is practised by barbers. Treatments take place in shops, in the home, and also on many street corners. It is a more vigorous style of massage than for women, designed to energize and stimulate. Sometimes manipulation is also involved. As with the women's tradition, different kinds of oils are used at different times of the year and to treat a range of different

conditions. Because of its cooling properties, coconut oil is often used in the summer, for example, while mustard oil may be preferred in the winter because it is warming. Being a head masseur is a fully recognized profession, and there is even a special caste attributed to it, in which the skills and expertise are handed down from father to son through each generation.

Experiencing an Indian head massage usually leaves the recipient feeling relaxed and unburdened. Some people even report a deep feeling of peace, such as may be experienced after meditation. Perhaps this is because the practice has its roots in India, where spirituality is so much an integral part of everyday life.

Combining the traditions

Traditional Indian head massage is somewhat different from the style of head massage that is generally practised in the West today. There are a number of reasons for this, although both styles of massage are equally effective and appropriate to the culture in which they are enjoyed.

head massage in India

Traditional Indian head massage is carried out in the context of a culture where social etiquette dictates that the masseur and recipient should be the same sex as one another. In India, a woman's hair is one of her most valuable beauty assets, and a great deal of time is devoted to cultivating the long, lustrous well-oiled locks that are so highly prized. The pace of life is unhurried and it is quite possible to spend several hours a week enjoying massage and beautifying rituals as a regular social activity. Personal grooming is carried out either in the home or the community, an excuse for friends, family and neighbours to gather together to exchange stories and catch up with one

▽ Massage is part of the everyday culture in Indian society and its benefits are increasingly appreciated by holidaymakers.

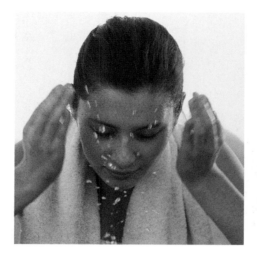

△ The trend in the West towards a faster lifestyle has meant that there is less time available for lengthy grooming procedures.

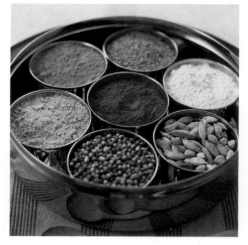

△ Traditional Indian head massage uses Ayurvedic oils from spices and plants, such as mustard, sesame, cinnamon, and cardamom.

another. Even when life is fast, the therapeutic value of massage is so much a part of everyday life that people still seem to find enough time to enjoy its simple and sensual pleasures.

the Western tradition

It is not so long ago in the West that practices such as hair-washing or bathing would also have taken up a large chunk of time each week. Today, however, the pace of life demands that grooming practices be as fast and practical as possible. In the Western world, the last fifty years or so has seen the accelerated development of a lifestyle based on speed, quantity and production. Showers, hairdryers and special beauty products, such as shampoos and conditioners "in-one", are designed to cater for our overriding need for speed and convenience, and a more perfunctory "wash-and-go" attitude towards personal maintenance has taken over.

redefining our values

This emphasis on speed and convenience means our primal need for touch is largely unmet, and there is a danger that living life in the fast lane is at the expense of a real

quality of life. Stress-related conditions are on the increase, and despite our material abundance many people experience a sense of emptiness. This has caused many Westerners to look for ways to discover their inner values and a more fulfilling lifestyle. The growing wave of interest in holistic

▽ The daily practice of yoga is part of the holistic Ayurvedic system of health, of which head massage is an integral component.

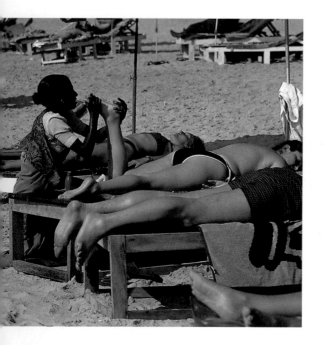

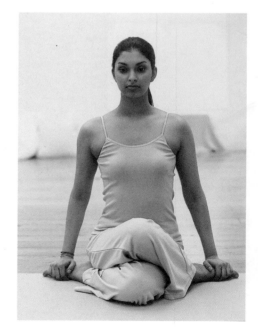

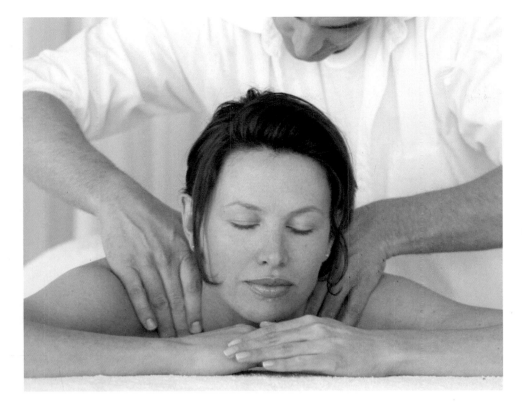

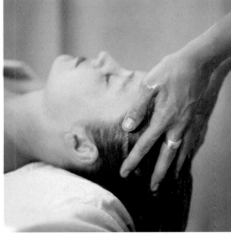

◁ As life continues to speed up, the need to slow down increases, and massage is increasingly being offered as a relaxation treatment in the Western beauty industry.

therapies, which take into account the emotional, mental and spiritual aspects of a person as well as the physical body, is part of this trend, with Indian head massage being just one of these.

a treatment for the modern world

Indian head massage is now finding and filling a niche in Western society. Gradually it has moved from being an "alternative" or "fringe" therapy to something that is becoming more widely recognized; many hairdressing salons now offer head massage as a service to their clients, for instance. However, the type of head massage being practised has been adapted to suit the constraints and demands of our culture.

Our work and lifestyle patterns have been changing, with the emphasis shifting away from physical activity to a more sedentary lifestyle. Every day we are confronted with huge amounts of information, which has to be processed, and we tend to live very active mental lives. Typically we suffer from mental overload, and because of our lack of physical activity, the resulting tension can get stuck in the body and emerge as discomfort.

▷ Massage is becoming increasingly mainstream and is recognized for its effective role in helping to get rid of stress and maintain balance.

Despite its name, the Western head massage routine includes more of the body than just the head. It also embraces the upper back, shoulders and neck, the main areas where we store tension in the body. While in India it is customary to use treatment oils on the hair and scalp, here head massage is done dry for the most part, although it is also possible to use oils for a special treatment every now and again. One of the great advantages of head massage (both Eastern and Western varieties) is that it is done clothes-on. This, together with its "dry" aspect, makes it highly versatile. Head massage can be carried out in a variety of

△ A head massage with oils is one of the most luxurious and relaxing treatments available for unwinding at the end of a day.

settings, both at home and in the workplace. Consequently, many massage practitioners are able to run a mobile service, travelling to people's homes or places of work to deliver head massage treatments for stress relief. It is important that the spiritual origins of head massage should not be forgotten, for it does much more than simply relieve physical tension. It also calms the spirit and helps to rebalance the body's own vital energies.

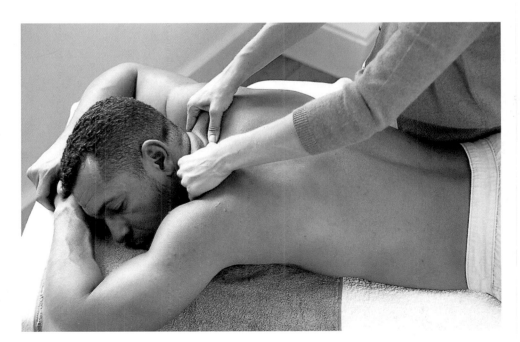

Body stress

The fast pace of modern life, combined with a sedentary lifestyle and an emphasis on mental activity, puts the body under a great strain. We can help to reduce body stress by practising certain stress-busting techniques and adopting healthy lifestyle habits. Because mind, body and spirit are part of one whole system, reducing stress in one area has a knock-on effect elsewhere. So techniques to relax the body also help the mind to unwind, while releasing pent-up emotions can help the body to relax.

a typical body profile

Many of us have a stressed body profile, with a "tension triangle" running from the top of the neck and down across the shoulders. The shoulders are often raised and hunched forward and the arms are gripped in tightly. This constricts the lungs and leads to shallow or restricted breathing. Poor posture throws the head out of alignment so that some muscles have to provide extra support for the skull's weight. As the back tightens this exerts pressure on the skull, pulling on the muscles at the base of the neck and around the head. This tightness is the most common cause of headaches and eyestrain,

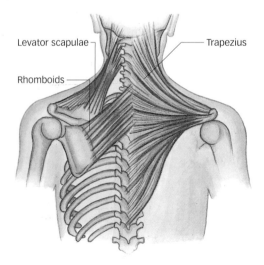

Levator scapulae — — Trapezius

Rhomboids —

△ Head massage works effectively to reduce tension in the upper body that accumulates over time, especially when a person is under stress or has a sedentary lifestyle.

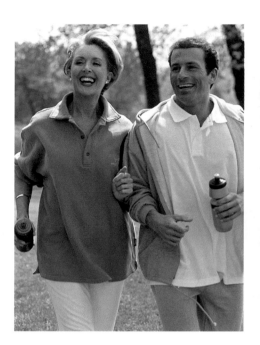

△ Regular exercise and movement, especially when done in the fresh air, is fundamental to a healthy, flexible, resilient body and to feeling and looking good.

as well as neck and shoulder pain. Tension may also show up in the lower back as the muscles there get shortened through lack of movement and poor posture.

using our muscles

Our muscles give the body strength and movement. To work effectively, they need a good balance between movement, exercise and relaxation. Holding the muscles in the same position for extended periods of time, such as when working at a computer terminal, makes them contract and shorten, impeding the circulation and flow of nutrients through the muscle fibre. This leads to muscle spasm and stiffness. Tired and contracted muscles are also more prone to injury, which is probably why conditions such as repetitive strain injury (RSI) and Carpal Tunnel Syndrome are becoming increasingly common.

To avoid overusing certain muscle groups at the expense of others, take a tip from yoga, where movements one way are always

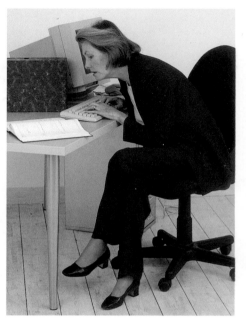

△ Sitting for long periods of time with your head turned to one side, such as when looking at a computer screen, or clipping the phone between your shoulder and ear, creates body stress.

balanced by a counter movement. So if you enjoy gardening, for example, intersperse bending over tasks, such as digging, with tasks that are performed standing up straight, like sweeping, or stretching up jobs, such as pruning tree branches.

Taking regular exercise is also one of the best stress-busting techniques. It relaxes your muscles, deepens your breathing, clears the mind and promotes restful sleep. Also, because it raises your endorphin levels (the "feel-good" chemical in the brain), it can lift your spirits and promote wellbeing. Find something that you enjoy, such as going to the gym, power walking, dancing, cycling or swimming. Even gentle stretching movements will help to discharge tension, keep the muscles toned and flexible and increase the body's range of movement.

emotional and mental stress

It is not only physical stress that impacts on the body. Emotional and mental pressures also contribute to body stress. When we are

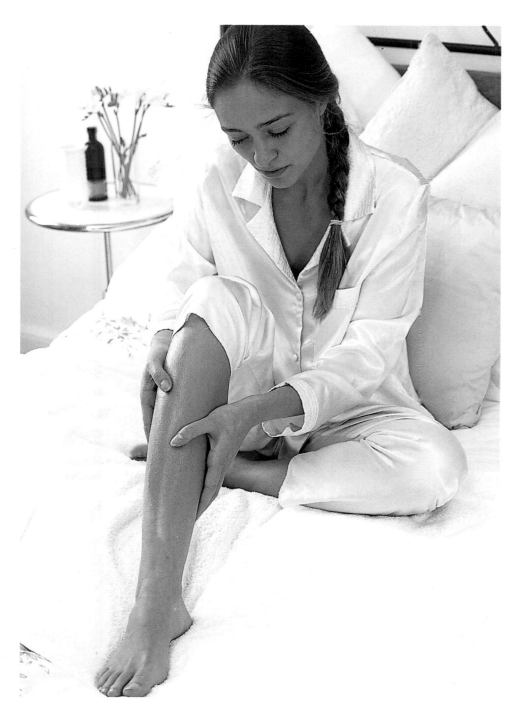

△ Taking time out to relax is essential for maintaining good health and wellbeing. Self massage is a nurturing way to do this, forcing you to sit down quietly.

extent that you may enter a very deep state of relaxation, akin to meditation, in which mind, body and soul are recharged.

food and drink

Our diet can either help or hinder our ability to cope with stress. Stimulants such as caffeine, alcohol and smoking deplete our nutritional store and contribute to stress levels. Sugary snacks and most processed foods stimulate the release of the stress hormone cortisol, leading to swings in blood sugar and energy levels. Opt instead for "slow release" energy found in whole foods – fresh fruits, vegetables, pulses and grains, seeds and nuts. Substitute herbal teas for tea and coffee and drink plenty of water to keep the body hydrated. Under stress the body uses up its nutrients more quickly, particularly the B vitamins, vitamin C, calcium and magnesium, so it's worth considering a multi-vitamin and mineral supplement to correct any deficiencies.

▽ Eating raw foods and drinking water helps reduce stressful thought patterns and is the best way to keep your body and skin hydrated.

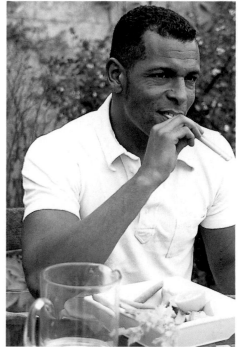

faced with a stressful situation, the body's first response is to activate its "fight/flight" response by pumping out adrenalin. This is nature's way of increasing our levels of alertness and ability to respond to danger – whether real or perceived – and causes physiological changes, such as rapid breathing, increased heartbeat, sweating and muscle tension. If the adrenalin that has been produced is not then utilized or discharged in some way it remains in the body, leading to high levels of anxiety and frustration as well as disturbances in thought processes and perception.

It can take a long time for the body to return to normal after having been aroused in this way, and ongoing stress can result in

exhaustion. At this stage, we may be continually tired and experience a range of unpleasant and frustrating physical and psychological symptoms.

relaxation and sleep

Being able to relax and enjoy a good night's sleep is one of nature's best stress cures. While we are under stress we need more sleep, but this is when we are most likely to experience sleep problems. Pursuits such as singing or painting, enjoying a long, warm aromatic bath, or eating delicious food, are all good ways of switching off in the evening. Massage is also excellent for relaxing body and mind. During a massage the brain waves can slow down to such an

The power of touch

On a physiological level, massage affects all the body systems, resulting in improved general functioning as well as relieving specific conditions. It can also assist with self-esteem, release emotional blocks, increase mental clarity, and help you to connect with your "inner light". Having a massage is simultaneously relaxing and refreshing. It is about taking time out to restore harmony and wellbeing so that you feel ready to take on the world again.

how massage works

The skin is the body's largest sensory organ. When it is touched, thousands of tiny nerve receptors on its surface send messages to the brain via the central nervous system. The brain interprets these messages and returns them to the muscles. Stroking can trigger the release of endorphins (the body's natural painkillers) and send messages of calm and relaxation. More vigorous massage works on the body's underlying muscles, easing tension and stiffness.

▽ **Massage contributes to our minimum daily touch requirements now recognized as fundamental to good health and wellbeing.**

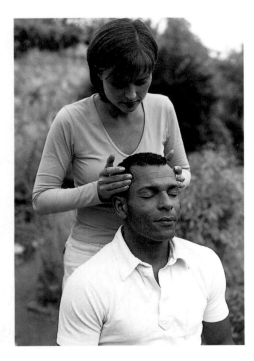

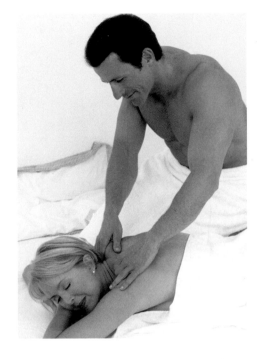

physical benefits

Relaxing massage causes the blood vessels and capillaries to dilate, which boosts the circulation and helps oxygenate the blood. This enables vital nutrients to be carried around the body more effectively, while temporarily reducing blood pressure and pulse rate. It also improves the appearance and quality of the skin. Massage stimulates

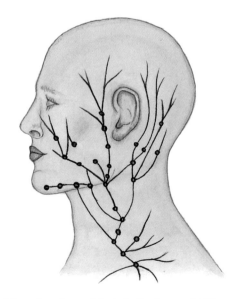

△ **Lymph nodes and ducts in the face and neck help eliminate toxins. Head massage stimulates the effectiveness of this cleansing action.**

◁ **Regular massage is a good immunity booster. Research has shown that it can have a protective effect on the body for up to a week after a single treatment.**

the functioning of the skin's sebaceous and sweat glands that work together to moisturize, clean and cool it. Massage also has an exfoliating action, helping to eliminate dead skin cells and thus resulting in a fresher appearance to the skin. Through boosting the circulation, head massage particularly helps to improve the condition of the hair and scalp by bringing the necessary nutrients needed for healthy hair growth. It can also help to relieve headaches, eyestrain, sinusitis, asthma and tension held in the jaw.

Massage also has a direct benefit on the body's muscular structure. By relaxing and stretching muscles that have become contracted and shortened with tension, massage helps the body to regain its flexibility as the elasticity and mobility of the body tissues is restored. These actions can help to ease painful muscles and improve posture by helping to bring the body's musculature back into a more balanced position. It can also help to restore muscles that have become weak and flaccid through underuse. The physical action of massage also works directly on the lymphatic system, helping the body eliminate lactic acid and other chemical wastes that contribute to pain and discomfort in the joints and muscles. Many lymphatic nodes are situated in the neck, back of the head, face and jaw.

As a massage treatment progresses and the body relaxes more deeply, there is a gradual switching over in body functioning towards the parasympathetic nervous system. This system operates outside of our conscious control and is related to the hidden work of general maintenance and repair and essential functions such as digestion and elimination. We are often in

▽ Blood is transported around the body by a complex network of arteries (shown in red) and veins (shown in blue). Massage increases peripheral circulation and assists blood flow through the system.

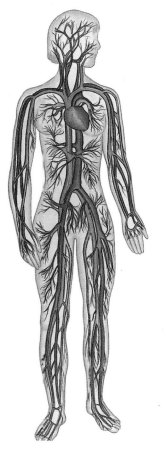

▽ Movement in the body is produced by the action of muscles. It is these skeletal muscles that register discomfort or ache when we get tired or put them under strain. Massage works directly on these key muscle groups.

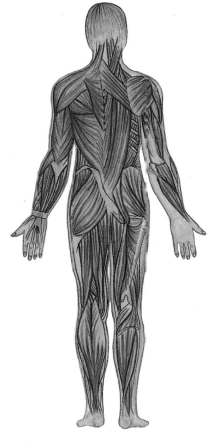

▽ Messages are transmitted between the brain and receptors and nerves through the body's "wiring system", which runs via the spinal cord. These include messages of relaxation from massage action.

so much of a rush that we don't give our bodies enough time for this important work. Massage is a good way of giving the body a "pit stop", where it can attend to its inner workings.

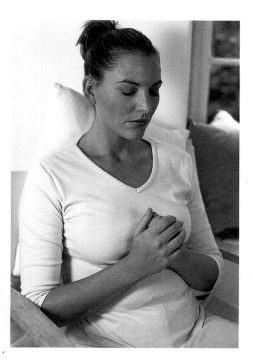

◁ Bright, sparkly eyes, glowing skin, relaxed muscle tone and an upright, balanced posture are some of the visible benefits of head massage.

mind and emotions

An extensive body of research supports the therapeutic claims of massage, with growing evidence that it can contribute to the relief of conditions such as stress, depression and anxiety. Head massage in particular has a significant impact on a mental level. The physical release of muscular tension and the increased blood supply to the head results in improved mental functioning and a greater sense of clarity. There is a reduction in mental exhaustion, feelings of irritability or being overwhelmed and a corresponding increase in alertness, mental agility, concentration and greater insightfulness.

Massage is also valued for its "feel-good" factor. As the body releases tension, a weight is lifted, leading to an increased sense of lightness and happiness. These emotional shifts correspond to the hormonal changes that occur in the body during a massage treatment. Research indicates that the level of stress hormones such as cortisol falls during massage, while the level of feel-good bonding hormones, such as oxytocin, significantly increases. Stress hormones have a weakening effect on the immune system.

nourishing the soul

Head massage also works on the energetic balance of the body through the chakra system, which centres around its spiritual dimension. By aligning body and soul through massage, a deep sense of peace, calm and balance can be achieved. The sense of lightness that people often feel after a treatment can also bring an increased awareness of their spiritual identity or inner light. After a massage people often feel more at one with themselves. Some people report an improved perspective on life, a return of their sense of humour, or say that they are simply more relaxed and comfortable within their own bodies.

Basic Techniques and Principles

It is not difficult to learn how to practise Indian head massage. By mastering a few basic strokes and techniques you will soon be on the way to becoming a proficient masseur. But although the strokes are important, they are not the only elements of a good massage. How you give the massage is equally important. Your ultimate aim is to give a treatment where all the strokes and techniques blend together, each flowing seamlessly from one to the next. To achieve this level of mastery takes a little practice.

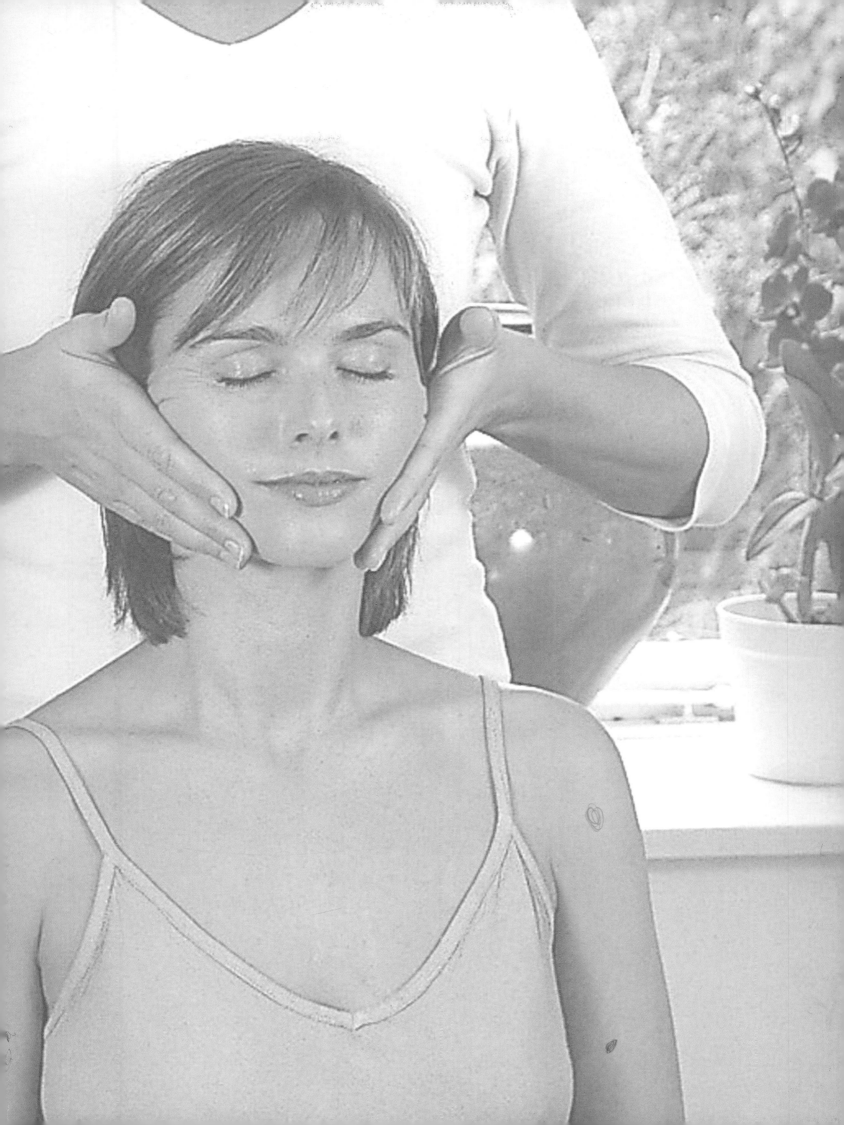

Basic massage strokes

Giving a head massage can be likened to playing music, with the basic strokes as the notes that are used to create the overall effect. Like musical notes, the strokes vary enormously, each one having its own particular quality and being used for different reasons to create different effects. The speed and depth with which you apply the strokes also affects how they come across.

stroking

One of the most basic and familiar massage strokes is stroking. It can be done with the hands, fingers or forearms over the head and body. Stroking has a calming and soothing effect on the nervous system, sending messages of relaxation to the brain via the skin's sensory nerve endings. Sometimes it connects to body memories of nurture and is a comforting, reassuring and affirming action. Strokes such as smoothing, ruffling, sliding or gliding are derived from stroking.

Stroking helps prepare the body for deeper massage work. It is also good after deep or vigorous actions such as pressure or kneading. This makes stroking a useful linking stroke to use in between different movements. It is also useful for travelling from one part of the body to another when working over different areas. This maintains contact with the body and keeps a sense of continuity. If you take your hands off the body or move away too quickly this disrupts the energetic flow and can feel strange for your partner.

friction strokes

Applied with the fingers and heel or sides of the hand, friction strokes use a rubbing or chopping motion. They are used on the head, shoulders and upper back and are vigorous and warming, stimulating the circulation and bringing heat and energy to the area being worked on. These strokes are useful for loosening muscle fibres and connective tissue that have become compacted with tension over a long time. Friction strokes feel exciting and energizing to receive, but some people also experience them as relaxing when done repeatedly.

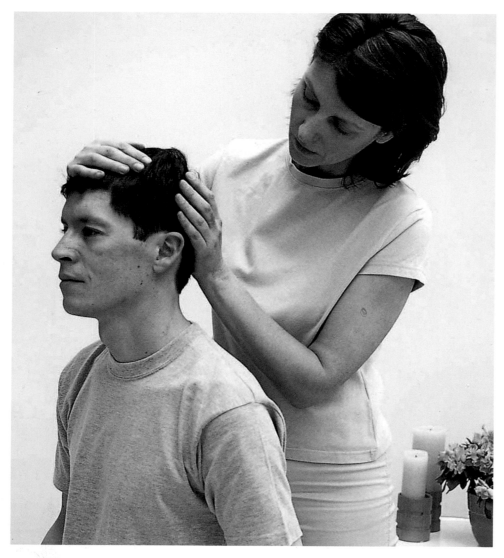

◁ For whole hand stroking, use the flat of your hand with your fingers pointing forwards and bring it slowly down over the back of the head. Let one hand follow the other in one flowing movement, and always support the head.

▽ Stroke over the upper body, shoulders or arms, working in a smooth and repetitive circular, zigzag, or back-and-forth action.

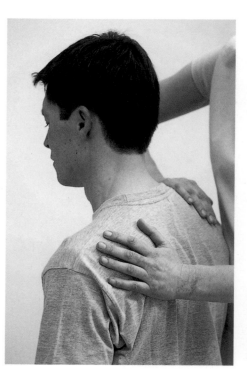

▷ Circular friction strokes with your thumbs will loosen tightness at the base of the neck and the tops of the shoulders. Begin in a small area, then make the circles wider as you work.

pressure strokes

Pressure strokes work in a number of ways. Sometimes the whole hand or forearm may be used to apply pressure, such as when pushing or pressing down on the shoulders or chest. These strokes work on releasing the body's deeper muscle layers. At other times, the fingers or thumbs are used to work on the body's energy system by applying pressure at specific release, or acupressure, points along the meridians (energy channels). When pressure is applied at such a point it helps to clear the energy channels so that the body's vital energies can flow freely. This helps to restore a sense of balance and equilibrium to the person.

Pressure points can be tender so your pressure needs to be firm but not cause undue pain. Gradually exert pressure on the points using your thumbs or fingers and hold it there for a few seconds before slowly releasing and moving on.

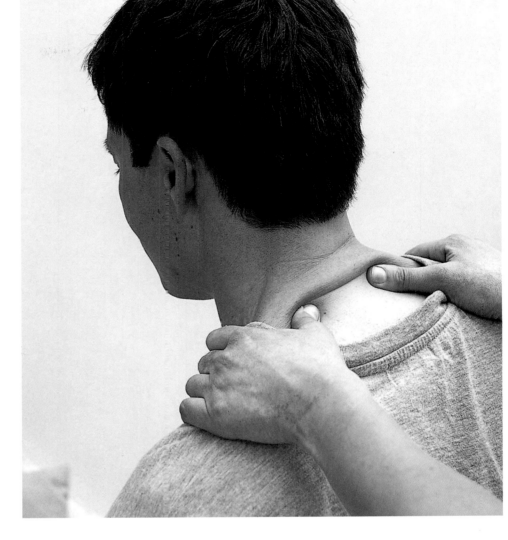

▽ Use firm pressure for friction strokes on the upper body, keeping your fingers straight but not rigid. Working rhythmically, you can build up momentum and massage at a fast pace.

▽ When doing friction strokes on the head, remember to support it with your other hand. Allow your own body to adjust and go with the momentum of the movement.

▽ When using pressure points on the delicate area of the face, when clearing sinus congestion for example, use your ring finger for the right amount of precise and responsive pressure.

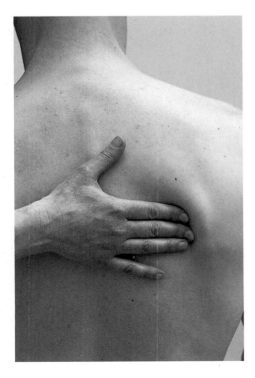
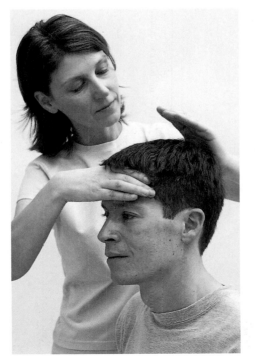
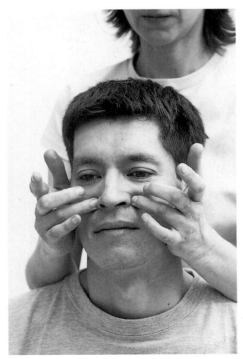

▷ When you do tapotement all over the scalp, as one hand rises let the fingertips of the other hand gently fall on the scalp .

tapotement

Also known as "percussion strokes" or "hacking", tapotement is a kind of tapping action. It is applied with the sides or tips of the fingers, and you can think of it as being a bit like playing a drum. One hand goes up as the other goes down. Tapotement is used on the head, the upper back and shoulders. This stroke works on the nervous and circulatory system. It has a stimulating effect and is light and refreshing to receive.

pulling and lifting

There is a range of strokes used in head massage that involve pulling, lifting, stretching and tugging. Most of these are done on the head itself, although some, such as lifting the shoulders, are also done on the body. They are done using the fingers and thumbs. These strokes work on the principle of tension followed by release, which leads to greater relaxation or increased mobility. As these strokes work in a lateral direction, that is away from the body, they also serve to direct and draw unwanted energies released by the massage, away from your partner's energy field.

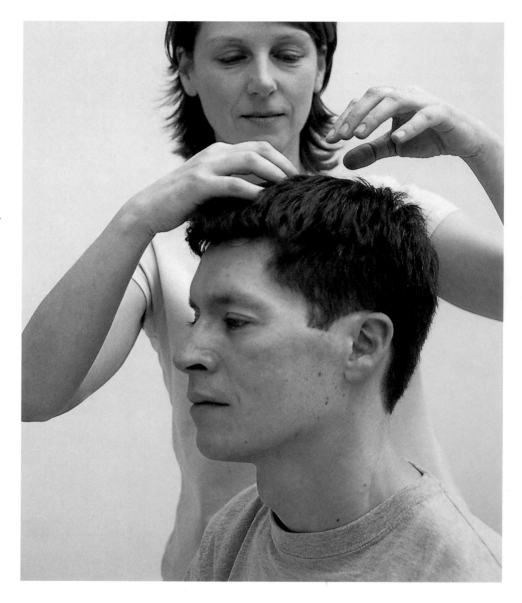

▽ When doing tapotement remember to keep your fingers soft as they land. Keeping your fingers spaced out a little will help with this.

▽ For a lifting action, gently pull your fingers to the very tips of your partner's hair. Let long hair fall through your fingers as you pull through.

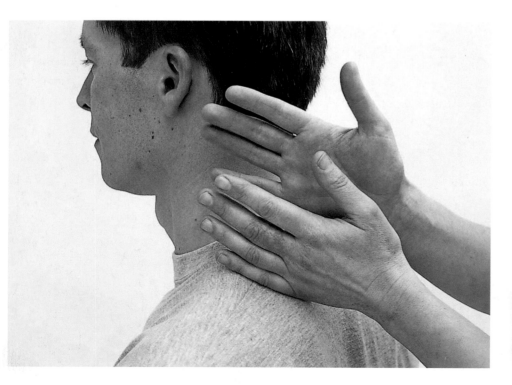

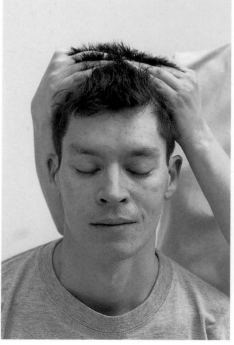

▷ When using a holding stroke, gradually let your hands descend on your partner and let them rest there in a relaxed and focused way for seven seconds or so.

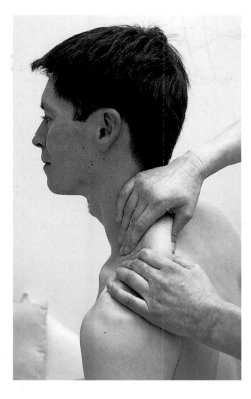

△ Knead the shoulders in a rolling action, not unlike working dough. Check the comfort level with your partner. If the shoulders are tight, reduce the pressure.

▽ When kneading in a small area such as under the chin, use a rolling action, working your fingers and thumbs together as you massage.

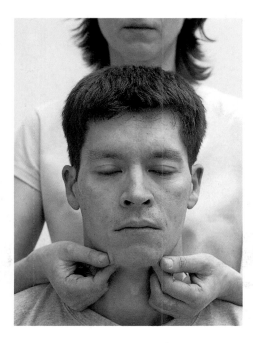

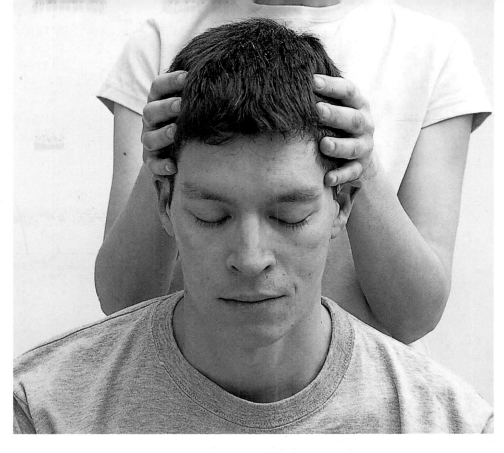

kneading and squeezing

The bread and butter of massage strokes are kneading and squeezing. In head massage these strokes may also be referred to as circling, rolling or pinching. Using the whole hands or thumbs and fingers, these strokes involve picking up the flesh away from the body and manipulating it in various ways. Kneading and squeezing strokes are appropriate for the more fleshy parts of the body such as the shoulders, the base and back of the neck, the chin and the outer edge of the ears.

holding

Although head massage is about movement, it is also about stillness. Holding involves keeping your hands still on your partner's head or shoulders, with a relaxed yet aware presence. It is often used to create a boundary around the session by marking its beginning and end. At the beginning, holding establishes initial contact with your partner and creates an energetic link between the two of you. It establishes communication through your hands, using massage as the language. At the end of the session it is a signal that the circle of energy between you and your partner is now complete and that you are about to move away. Holding can ground the treatment by holding the energy, and give healing, love, and energy to your partner.

key principles

There are a number of principles to keep in mind. The first is to stand at a comfortable distance from your partner when you work, not too close and not too far away. This is so that you can get a good leverage and your partner can feel your reassuring presence.

Second, stay as relaxed as you can and do not hold yourself tense or rigid. You need to be like a dancer, having your feet on the floor yet allowing your movements to be free and flowing.

Third, tune into and be sensitive to your partner's changing energies and moods through the different phases of the massage.

It may take a little practice and trust before you feel confident enough to be able to pick up and respond to the subtle nuances. If your partner is ticklish, omit stroking and light touches and instead use the flat of your hand, a firmer touch and work at a lower speed. Try and enjoy yourself, as how you are feeling will be communicated to your partner through your hands.

Cautions and contraindications

Indian head massage is one of the safest types of massage and can be practised on just about anyone. As with any therapy, though, it is important to be aware that there are certain situations where you should be particularly careful or where a treatment may be contraindicated. If ever you are in doubt, always err on the side of caution and ask a doctor or professional therapist for advice before giving a treatment.

At the beginning of the session, ask your partner how they are feeling, and check out if they have any medical conditions and/or are taking any medication. You should also check for any recent injuries, fractures or surgery, particularly in the head or upper body area. If your partner is feeling unwell,

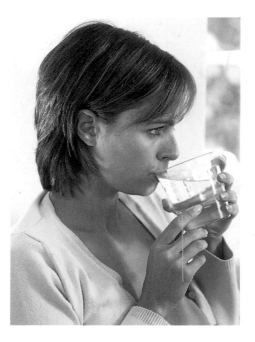

△ Drinking a glass of water is a good way to begin and end a massage treatment, as it is cleansing and grounding for the system.

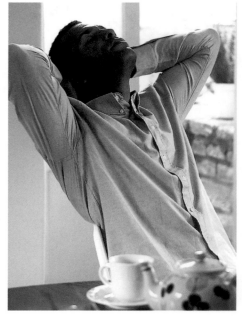

△ If your partner is particularly tense, and their muscles are sore and tender, always make sure you massage with caution in order not to aggravate their discomfort.

▽ Make sure you take enough to time talk through the massage with your partner to establish a rapport and sort out any concerns.

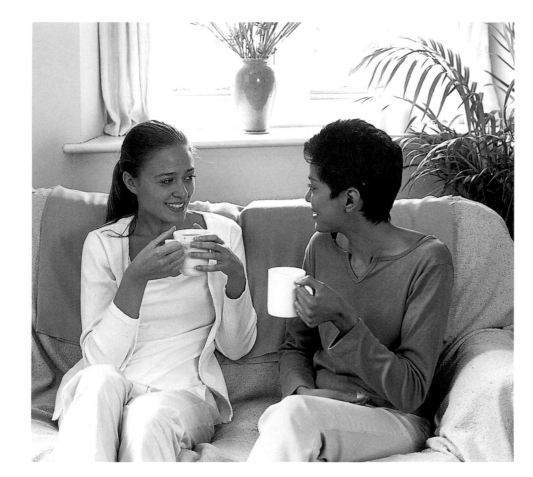

it is best to postpone the treatment, as it could aggravate their condition. This could include a cold, a temperature, any acute infectious disease or skin conditions.

skin conditions

Be aware of any cuts, bruises, open sores, blistering, redness or swelling. These areas will be painful when touched and could become infected, so are best avoided. Any contagious skin conditions, such as ringworm, impetigo, scabies or herpes (cold sores), should also be avoided to prevent the risk of you picking up the infection.

Ringworm is a fungal infection. It begins as small red papules that spread to form red, itchy, shiny circles under the skin over the body. Impetigo is a highly contagious bacterial skin condition, usually found around the mouth, nose and ears, in which raised, fluid-filled sores seep and leave honey coloured crusts on the skin. Scabies is identified by small reddish marks around the wrist and in between the fingers, and is

▷ During times of illness it is inadvisable to massage deeply, although a tender loving touch can be so comforting and healing – to give as well as to receive.

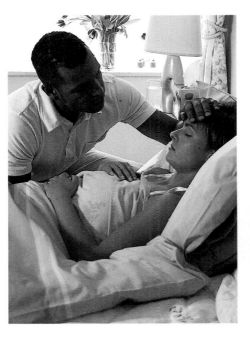

extremely itchy. Herpes is a viral infection that erupts in sores around the mouth and nose, particularly after exposure to the sun or during times of stress.

While eczema and psoriasis may look unsightly they are not contagious. Unless the skin is broken, they are not contra-indicated for massage. However it is best to check with your partner that they find it comfortable to be touched in these areas.

Scalp conditions to be aware of include head lice (nits), ringworm and folliculitis. The latter is a bacterial infection with swelling and pain around the hair follicles.

the skeleton

Conditions relating to the bones and the skeleton, which include brittle bones, osteoporosis and spondylitis, are clearly contraindicated for massage because of the high risk of injury to your partner.

You should also be aware of any head, neck or shoulder injuries, such as whiplash. Head massage could make these conditions worse, so check with a doctor.

circulatory problems

With high blood pressure there could be a risk of clotting so always seek medical advice. When this is related to high stress levels, massage can be very effective in reducing stress triggers, but do seek medical advice first. Low blood pressure increases the likelihood of feeling faint so make sure your partner gets up slowly after the massage. Recent haemorrhages, a history of thrombosis and embolisms are other blood disorders that can cause problems. Anyone with any one of these conditions should not be massaged in the absence of medical supervision.

epilepsy

Although epilepsy is normally controlled and stabilized by medication, it is thought that stimulating massage, particularly to the head, can trigger an attack, although it may

be possible to massage the upper back, shoulders and arms. This condition needs medical advice before treatment.

cancer

Massage is contraindicated with cancer but it is increasingly recognized as having a supportive role in palliative care. Always seek medical advice first. It is inadvisable to massage immediately after chemotherapy or radiation treatment.

pregnancy

Head massage is an ideal treatment during pregnancy, as the woman can remain sitting

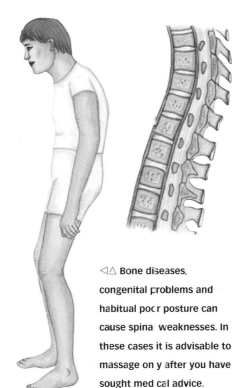

◁△ Bone diseases, congenital problems and habitual poor posture can cause spinal weaknesses. In these cases it is advisable to massage only after you have sought medical advice.

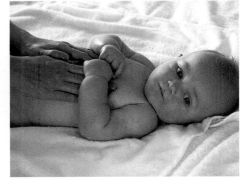

△ As babies' skulls are so delicate, due to the unfused fontanelles, massaging the head is inadvisable, but gentle baby body massage with oils is a nurturing alternative.

rather than having to lie down which can be awkward and uncomfortable. Remember that you are treating two people, not one, so be particularly sensitive. Use a lighter pressure than normal, particularly during the first trimester.

children and the elderly

The rule of working lightly also applies to children, the frail and the elderly. Adjust your pressure to the energy of the person you are massaging. Even when treating robust-looking older children, it is advisable to work lightly until you are both familiar with massage. If it is done too strongly it can stimulate a rise of energy that is too much for your partner's young body and could cause them to faint.

emotional response

Sometimes people can have emotional reactions to massage such as feeling tearful or upset. This is because unexpressed feelings seem to remain locked in the body and the effect of massage can be to release them. In these situations, be sensitive in responding to your partner. It is a good idea to ask them if they would like you to continue or to pause before carrying on.

Getting started

One of the beauties of Indian head massage is that it can be performed almost anywhere and doesn't need a lot of equipment. The essentials are a suitable chair, a pair of hands, a willing heart and knowledge of what to do. To get the most out of it, a few preliminaries will help put you and your partner in the right frame of mind. These include getting all your equipment together, scene setting, and preparing yourself and your partner for a treatment.

seating

The best chair is one without any arms and a relatively low back to give you easy access to your partner. Cushions or pillows can be used to soften or raise seating or to provide comfort or support. However, you can always adjust the massage according to the situation. For instance, if you can't get to your partner's arms easily then just stroke them gently. If your partner is too tired to sit up, they could sit astride the seat and lean

▽ **Make sure that you prepare a relaxing space and have everything to hand before you begin so that your massage will go smoothly. A low backed chair without arms is ideal.**

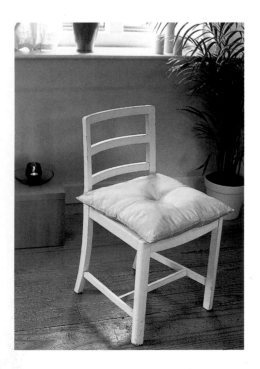

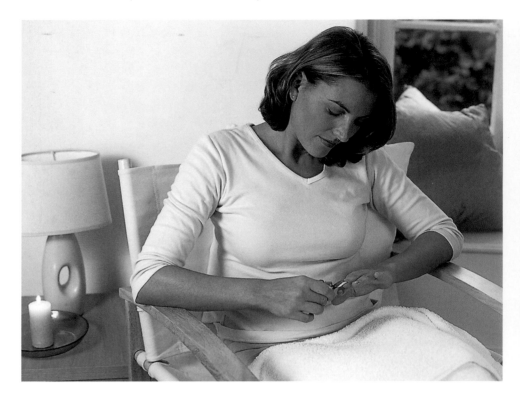

over the back of the chair, supported by cushions. The most important thing is for them to be comfortable.

preparation

Clean and tidy the room to create a harmonious space that is easy to work in. Make sure that it is warm, and eliminate as many potential distractions as you can. Unplug the phone, turn off any mobiles, and put a "do not disturb" sign on the door.

Next think about mood setting. Sound, lighting and fragrance can all be used to help create a particular ambience and turn the room into a healing space. Candles give a soft and subdued light, while certain types of music can help you relax. Burning incense or vaporizing essential oils will fragrance the air, as well as helping to clear impurities. If you want to use music and/or scent, choose something that both you and your partner will enjoy.

Make sure that you are wearing loose comfortable clothes, and take a few moments to make the following preparations. You also need to take a few

△ **Remove your watch, and any rings or bracelets, and wash your hands. File your nails so that they are short and smooth to the touch.**

▽ **Make sure your hair is tied back or clipped up so that it does not fall over your face as you massage, as this is distracting.**

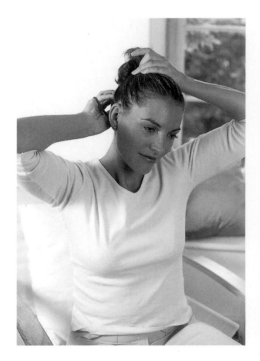

▷ Spend some talking with your partner so you can check for contraindications as well as tune in to each other and establish a smooth rapport before beginning the session.

equipment

If you are using any oils, set them out with a little bowl for mixing. You will also need a pack of tissues for wiping your hands and a blanket to cover your partner if they get cold. Also have plenty of drinking water available for yourself and your partner.

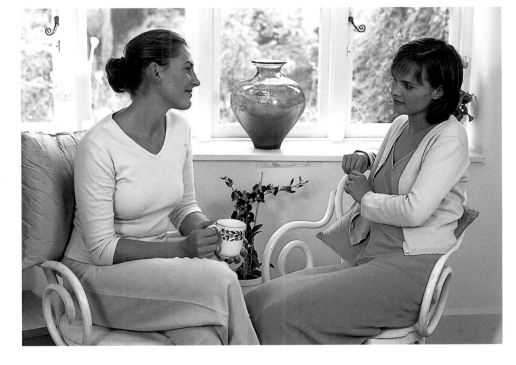

moments to make sure you are "grounded". To do this, sit in a comfortable chair and relax. Now close your eyes and take a deep, slow breath into your belly. As you breathe out, imagine channels of energy travelling down through your body, legs and feet and into the ground. Think of your feet having extensions that stretch deep down into the earth like the roots of a tree. As you breathe in, imagine the energy coming up again through the roots and into your body, replenishing you with new energy. As you

▽ Take some time to breathe deeply, relax your own mind and body and tune in and calm yourself, otherwise known as grounding.

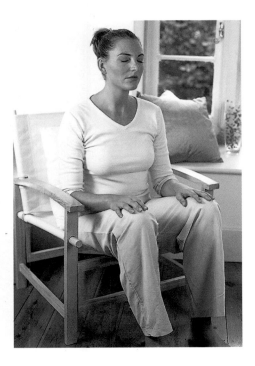

breathe in and out see this continuous movement of energy. Once you are grounded, you are ready to warm up.

warming up

Giving yourself a shake-out will warm up your body and help you let go of tension. Stand in a clear space and have a chair to lean on if necessary. Pick up one leg and shake it out so that it wobbles. Circle your foot at the ankle in both directions. Repeat on the other side. Next move to your arms and repeat. Circle your hands at the wrists in both directions and shake them out.

making contact and tuning in

Sit with your partner and spend a few moments checking in together, making sure there are no contraindications. Review any areas of tension and find out where they would like you to prioritize. Have them remove any jewellery and loosen their hair if necessary. It is best if they are wearing a loose t-shirt or vest top. Make sure they are sitting comfortably, with both feet placed squarely on the ground. You might like to put a pillow under their feet for comfort. Ensure there is enough space for you to work around them freely. Ask your partner if they will let you know if there is anything they don't like or is uncomfortable during the massage, and give them permission to relax their body and mind and switch off during the treatment. You are now ready to tune in to your partner.

Stand behind your partner and place your hands on top of their head. Close your eyes and let go of your thoughts, tuning in to your partner's breathing and energy field. If you have a spiritual belief, you might offer it up as a type of prayer. Then very gently move your partner's head, first forwards and then backwards, and then to the right and left. Finally, let your hands slide lightly down from the head, over the neck to a point level with the bottom of the shoulder blades. You are now tuned in and ready to begin.

▽ The beginning of a massage always begins with a non-verbal tuning-in as your hands touch the head and your energies merge.

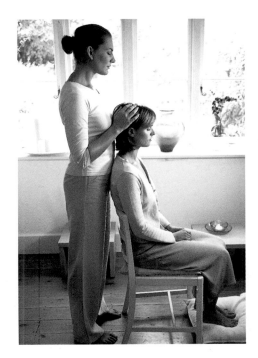

Head massage with a partner

Once you have made all the necessary preparations and have spent a few moments tuning in with your partner, you are ready to begin giving a head massage treatment. The following pages give detailed instructions for a sequence of movements using the basic strokes. To help you, this sequence is divided into sections, each relating to the area of the body being worked on. It begins with the upper back.

the upper back

The strokes outlined here help to relax and release tension in the upper back. Many aches and pains, including tension headaches, begin in this area, particularly in the trapezius (the large muscles over the back of the neck and shoulders). Never work directly on the spine.

▽ **1** Place your thumbs in the ridge that runs up either side of the spine at a point roughly parallel to the bottom of the scapulae (shoulder blades). Spread your other fingers on the back to support your thumbs. To increase your leverage and to prevent back strain, you may need to take a step backwards or bend your knees as you do this stroke.

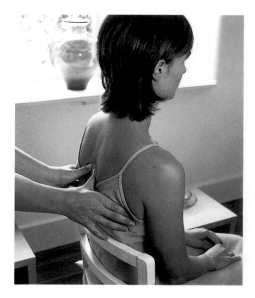

△ **2** In an upward movement, slide and push your thumbs up on either side of the spine. Continue up the back and neck to the top of the spine at the base of the skull. Go back to the starting position and repeat three times, increasing the pressure with each movement. This stroke helps release tension in the muscular attachments that run up the back.

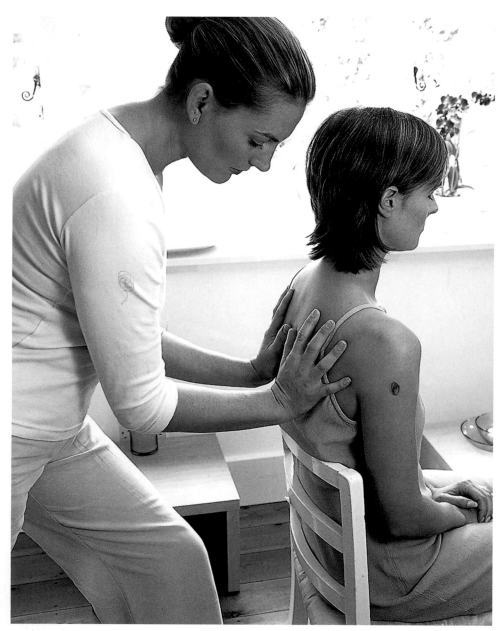

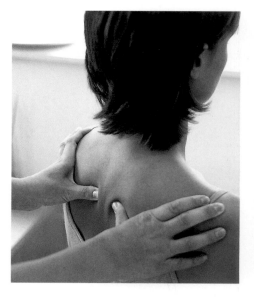

△ **3** Find the muscles that run up either side of the spine, about 2cm (¾in) out. You can feel their line with your fingers, like a rope or a cord down the side of the spine. Using your thumbs or the small bony part on the outside edge of the wrist, make small circular strokes on the belly of the muscle. Work from the middle of the back up to the shoulders.

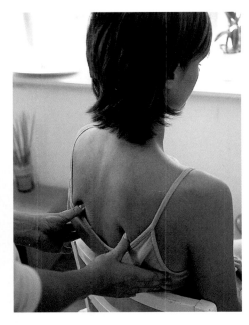

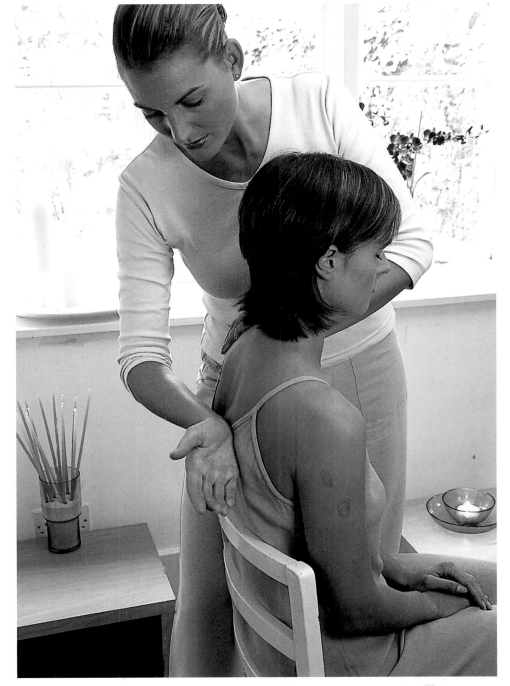

△ **4** Place both your thumbs at the bottom outside edge of your partner's scapulae. Push and slide your thumbs in an upward direction, moving along the edge of the scapulae all the way round to the top of the shoulders. Sweep round to your starting point and repeat three times. This helps release the trapezius attachments around the scapulae.

▽ **5** Move to the left side of your partner and place your left hand gently on their shoulder. Position the fingertips of the first two fingers of your right hand at the base of your partner's right scapula. Using a fast jabbing motion move your fingertips back and forth in a friction movement against or underneath the outer edge of the scapula. Work upwards to the outside edge where the arm attaches and repeat two more times. The most vigorous of the strokes described here, this action releases tension in the muscle attachments and layers.

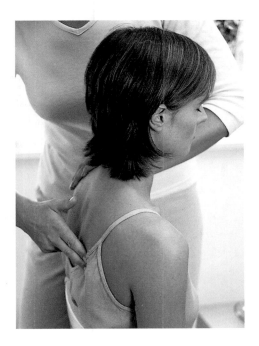

△ **6** Follow the same path around the edge of the scapula, this time using the side of your hand and wrist. Place the side of your hand and the small bony ridge of your wrist at the base of the scapula. Using a circular movement, as if drawing little circles, follow around the edge of the scapula as you progress in an upward direction. This stroke helps to flatten and smooth out the muscles. Repeat three times.

▷ **7** From the top of the scapula stroke the whole shoulder joint in a wide generous movement, using the whole of your hand. Make the circles increasingly wide to take in more and more of the upper back. This is a calming action after the vigorous strokes earlier on. Once you have finished move round to stand at the other side of your partner and repeat steps 5–7 on the other side.

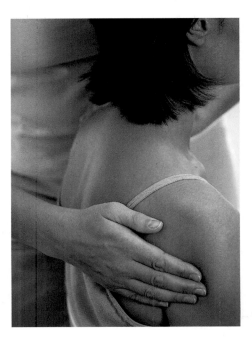

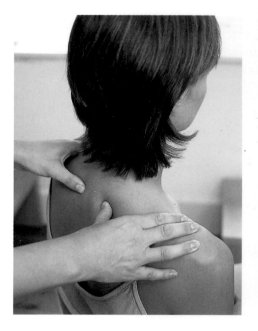

shoulders and arms

After the upper back, the next part of the massage sequence is to work on the shoulders and arms. When you get to this part of the massage, most people are usually very grateful as the arm and shoulder area is generally very tight and achy. Our arms perform countless tasks that we take for granted – pushing, pulling, lifting and carrying all manner of things, big and small. Shoulder tension is also connected with emotional burdens and responsibilities from "carrying the world on our shoulders".

When massaging the shoulders, it is best to proceed cautiously as the muscles can have a tendency to contract even further, particularly in response to deeper massage. If you feel this happening then change immediately to lighter, more sweeping strokes.

▽ **1** Rest your hands lightly on your partner's shoulders and as they breathe out use your body weight to gently push down on their shoulders. Notice with your hands when you feel the resistance and release. Next use both hands to make a wide sweeping movement, brushing across the tops of the shoulders away from the body. Do this a few times. It is a gentle stroke that warms up the area and prepares the body for deeper massage.

△ **2** Rest your thumbs at the base of your partner's neck. Using the pads of your thumbs make circular, pressing stokes over the whole of the trapezius muscle that runs along the base of the neck, top of the back and across the shoulders. This warms up the muscles and makes them more pliable for kneading. How hard you press will depend on the feedback you receive from your partner.

▽ **3** Pick up a roll of flesh from the trapezius muscles with the thumb and fingers of one hand and slide it across to feed the other hand in a smooth rhythmical way. Repeat the movement with the other hand. This kneading action is similar to kneading bread dough. Keep this up for a few minutes and establish a regular rhythm, adjusting the speed and pressure according to your partner's needs. This is a very popular stroke for a key area of tension. Work for a few minutes on each shoulder without overworking the muscles.

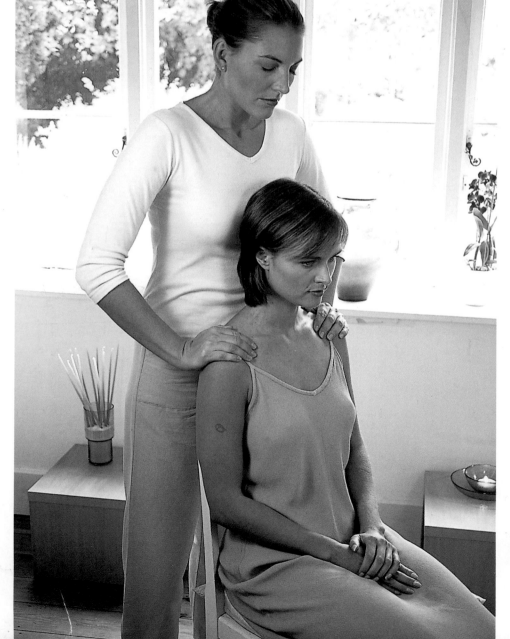

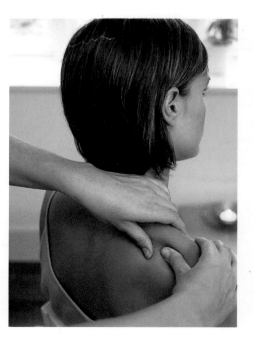

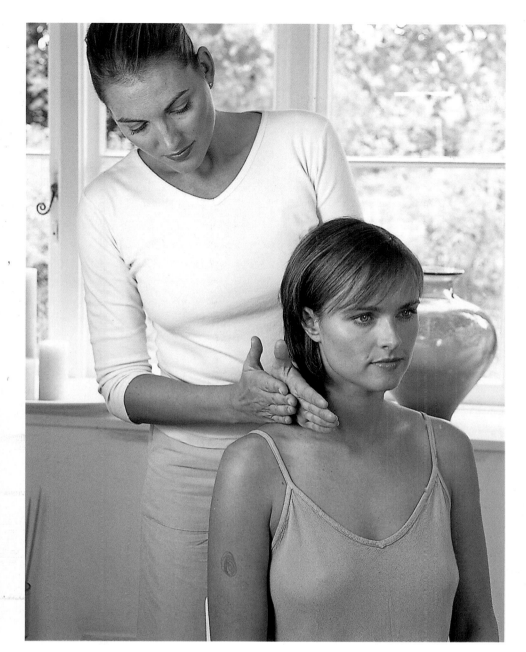

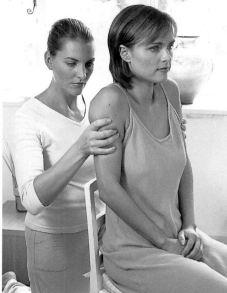

△ **6** Slide your hands down to the tops of your partner's arms and hold there for a moment in preparation for the shoulder shrug. Ask your partner to take a deep breath in and as they do so lift their arms slightly so that their shoulders are raised near their ears. As they breathe out, let go of their arms. The shoulders may drop down abruptly. Repeat once.

▽ **7** Place the heel of each hand at the top of your partner's arms. Roll down the arms, turning your wrists in a circular action. Use firm pressure as you go and continue down to the elbow joint. In a continuous movement, roll around to the back of the arm and move back up. Roll over the tops of the shoulders and continue down the arms again until you have completed the whole cycle three times.

△ **4** Place both hands together as if in prayer position and put them side-on near the base of your partner's neck. Slowly rub your hands together, applying a little pressure as you move across the surface of your partner's shoulder in a sawing action. Build up speed as you get into the rhythm of it. Travel across the top of one shoulder and saw down a little into the upper back area, working on the muscles either side of the spine. Then in a continuous movement, jump your hands over the spine and continue working on the opposite side of the upper back, travelling up and across to the other shoulder. Repeat three times.

▷ **5** Lift and drop your hands alternately. As each one descends, let the sides of your fingers hit down lightly on the skin for this hacking stroke. Your fingers should be soft as they knock together on impact. Move across the shoulders and upper back, building up momentum. Work over the area three times. Slow down gradually to bring to a close.

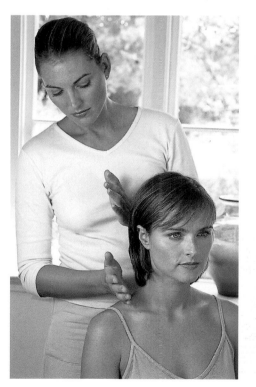

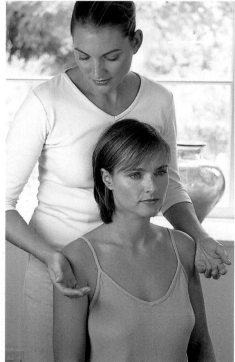

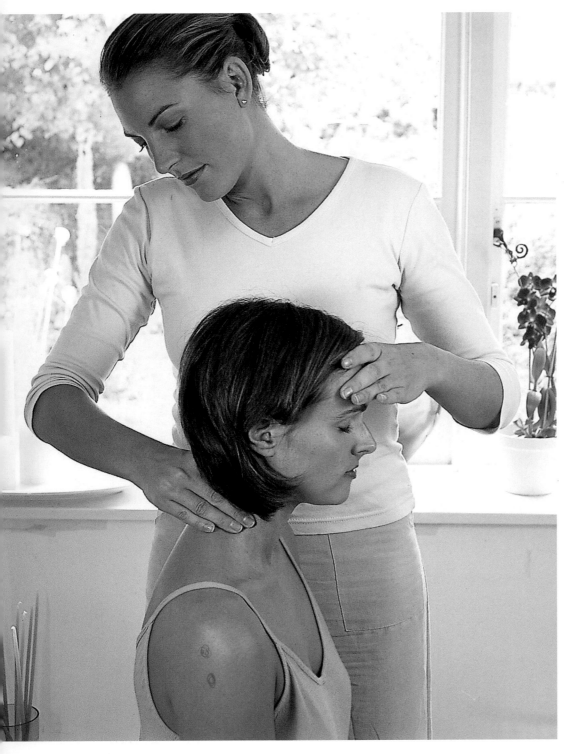

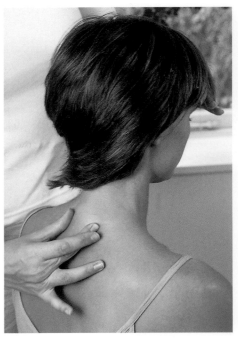

◁ **1** Stand to the left of your partner. To support your partner's head, place your thumb and middle finger of your left hand on either side of their forehead, using a firm but soft grip. Place your right hand at the base of the neck and with a wide span, grasp and pull back the neck's flesh and muscles. Sweep your hand up a little and repeat the movement in the middle and at the top of the neck. Repeat the whole sequence three times. This warms up the neck and loosens the muscles.

the neck

The head, neck and back are held in dynamic relationship. When all three are working as they should, we tend to feel good in every respect. The neck has a particularly important part to play. It should be long, stretching up and away from the shoulders, supporting the head with a wide range of movement. Poor posture and stress cause tension in the neck, the muscles to become imbalanced and the head to be thrown forward. Due to the uneven strain, some neck muscles can be in a permanent state of contraction, with tension knots particularly at the base and top of the neck. This imbalance

puts a tremendous strain on the upper back and shoulder muscles because they are part of the same muscle group. Over time this can build up and become chronic, making the neck more prone to injury. Tight neck muscles are one of the main causes of tension headaches.

Massaging the neck helps to ease out tension and stiffness, giving greater comfort and increased mobility. It can also help to relieve headaches. When working on the neck you need to support your partner's head with one hand. Swap hands as often as you need to, but keep the movement flowing. Make sure you work at a level that is comfortable for your partner.

△ **2** Continuing to support your partner's head with your left hand, use your right thumb to slide up the muscles, massaging in a circling action. Continue to the top of the neck where the skull attaches. Bring your thumb down and repeat. Follow with some circular strokes (petrissage) around the back and sides of the neck, using your fingers and thumbs together in a circling upward movement. Do not go as far round to the front as the windpipe or cause your partner any discomfort.

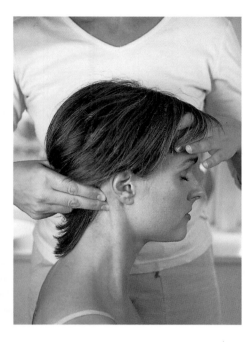

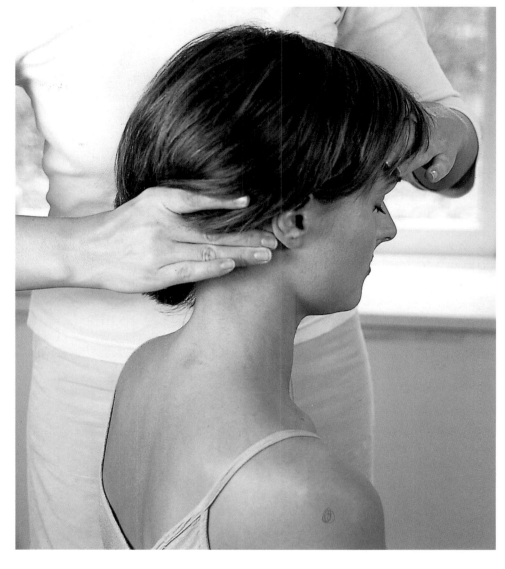

△▽ **3** Starting at the bony ridge behind the back of the ear, make small circular strokes across the base of the skull to the middle of the neck, using the first two fingers of your right hand. Continue the stroke down the middle of the neck along the ridge by the side of the spine. Repeat three times. Work very sensitively, as this area is often tender. Gently increase the pressure as the neck muscles release. Swap hands, move to your partner's right side and repeat steps 2–3.

△ **4** Stand on your partner's left and, supporting their head (step 1), stretch out your right hand to reach either side of the base of their skull with your thumb and middle finger. Press and slide your outstretched fingers along the base of the skull to the middle and then move down the neck on either side of the spine. Repeat three times. This stroke works on the lymphatic system and helps flush out toxins released earlier. The hand position is good when using your thumb to work on pressure strokes to the neck.

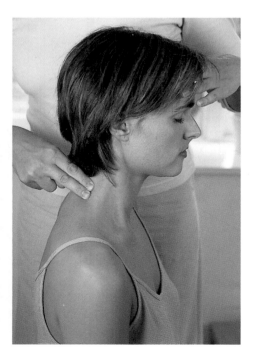

pressure strokes for the neck

As you perform this massage routine, you will be stimulating acupressure points that can have a therapeutic influence on specific body organs and systems and help relieve symptoms of ill health. It can also release endorphins, serving to unblock stuck energies and restore balance to the body as a whole. When massaging over these points, be sensitive to the amount of pressure you apply. Exerting pressure on the various points around the neck can help stiffness and pain, headaches, eyestrain and imbalances in the eyes, ears and throat. Massage here will also have a positive effect on relieving stress, exhaustion and irritability. In the case of pregnancy avoid pressure strokes to the neck and shoulders.

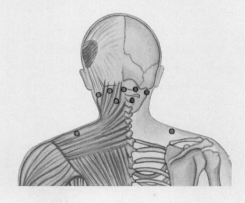

the face

Facial expressions and "character" lines can tell us a lot about someone. Our facial muscles are highly versatile and work hard in transmitting – or concealing – information about ourselves. From a young age, we learn how to "pull ourselves together" or to put on a "brave face" to avoid showing certain emotions. This results in tension being stored in the facial muscles and is compounded by the stress of ordinary living. Typically, worry lines develop across the forehead, the jaw is clenched tight and the eyes can assume a hard, staring look, even appearing to stand out of their sockets.

Because of the very high number of nerve receptors on the facial skin's surface, face massage is a mainline to relaxation. It not only helps the muscles let go of tension, but also sends relaxing signals to the brain, which are then transmitted to the rest of the body.

Facial expressions can be part of our protective armour, and people can look much more youthful and open after a massage because defensiveness has been dropped, and the face restored to a state of natural relaxation.

△ **1** Stand behind your partner and softly draw your hands down over their face to cup the bottom of the face at the jaw. Then slowly draw your fingers and palms up over the face, trailing them across the cheeks and up to the tops of the ears. Extend this stroke to sweep over the eye sockets and take in the forehead. Repeat this upward movement a few times.

▽ **2** Return your hands to cup the bottom of the face, and place the thumb and index finger of both hands in the middle of the chin. With your thumbs on top and the index fingers underneath, gently pick up the fold of flesh along the chin and roll it between your fingers. Work along and just under the edge of the jaw line towards the ears. Repeat three times.

location of the lymph nodes

Part of the body's immune system, the lymphatic system plays a key part in eliminating toxins. The lymph nodes make and store white blood cells and process wastes and bacteria before passing fluids back into the circulatory system. Fluids are delivered to the nodes via ducts located throughout the body. The ducts depend on suction and muscle pumping to work effectively, and they have one way valves. Without bodily movement to trigger its mechanisms, its functioning can become sluggish and impaired. An increase in pollution and toxins, compounded by today's sedentary lifestyles, can often result in the lymphatic system becoming overloaded. Massage action can stimulate the effective functioning of the lymph. Face massage works directly on the lymph nodes located in the face and neck and can directly support and benefit detoxing.

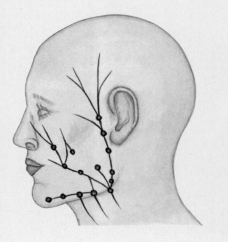

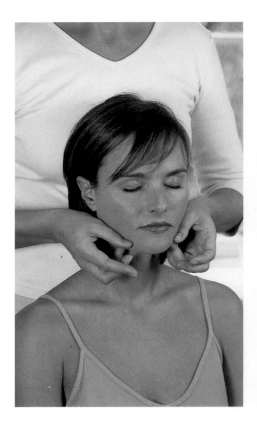

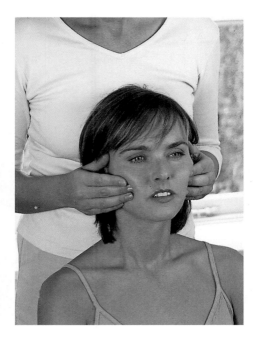

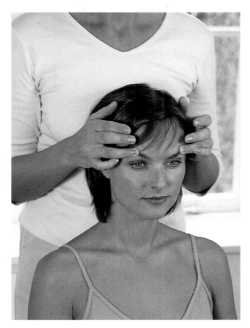

△ **3** At the jaw socket by the ears, make circular strokes with your fingertips, paying particular attention to the hinge area. If your partner is holding their jaw tight, you may be able to feel it release and drop as you work. You could also ask them to drop their mouth open which will help release jaw tension.

△ **4** Use your ring fingers to gently press at three evenly spaced points along the eyebrow. Begin at the inner edge and finish at the outer. Repeat the stroke directly above these points in the middle of the forehead and then at top of the forehead. Repeat the sequence two times. Finish by stoking the forehead.

the ears

In Chinese medicine, the ears are seen as a microcosm of the whole body, rather like the feet in reflexology. The earlobe corresponds to the head and the face areas, the outside edge to the spine, and the middle to the body's inner organs. In such a small surface area, the ear is highly concentrated in acupressure points. Massage to the ears can stimulate the brain, improve the movement of lymph, help circulation and alleviate pain and stiffness generally from the muscles and joints.

The ears are full of nerve endings and their massage can feel wonderfully pleasant, intimate and stimulating for the recipient. When massaging use your fingers and thumbs to work along the outside edge, and only use your index or ring finger to trace inside the hollows of the ear because it is so sensitive here. Work both ears simultaneously, and use your fingers to twiddle along the outer edge or gently pull down on the ear lobes. A calming way to end a massage is to cover your partner's ears with the palms of your hands for a few moments.

▽ The ear has a high concentration of pressure points, and according to Chinese medicine can be seen as a mircrocosm of the entire body.

location of the sinuses

Structurally the sinuses are four air-filled pockets situated in the skull and in the face. These cavities are lined with a mucous membrane that often gets inflamed, which can range from the low-level discomfort of a stuffed-up nose to a more serious and painful infection. Face massage can help relieve discomfort in the cheeks and forehead, reduce pressure around the eyes and clear stuffed-up noses caused by a sinus condition. Its soothing action can also help alleviate strong emotional states associated with sinusitis, such as stress and worry, irritation, guilt and grief. These states can cause tension in the chest contributing to the closing up of the sinus passages.

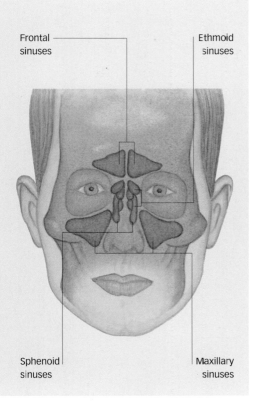

Frontal sinuses — Ethmoid sinuses

Sphenoid sinuses — Maxillary sinuses

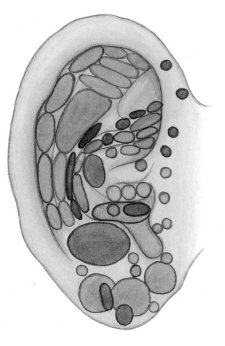

the head

The final part of the massage sequence is spent working on the head, which contains many pressure points that relate to other parts of the body. People are often surprised by how much tension is stored in the musculature of the head. This may be related to tension held in the back muscles travelling up the spine and into the head, or it may be caused by mental overload. Massaging the head is a very effective antidote to stress, as it loosens tension in the scalp and benefits the whole body.

Keep your hands moving as you use the several different strokes, keeping a sense of rhythm and flow as one stroke moves into the next. As you start each different stroke, begin slowly, building up the pace before slowing it down again as you draw to a close and move to the next movement.

▽ **1** Stand to the left of your partner and support their forehead. Put the right hand at the front of their face before the ear by the hairline. Using three or four fingers, rub the scalp briskly back and forth in a vigorous sawing movement. This is known as the "windscreen wiper" stroke. Work from the front of the head down to the hairline at the back, moving across the whole of the left side of the head. Do this three times, then repeat on the other side of the head.

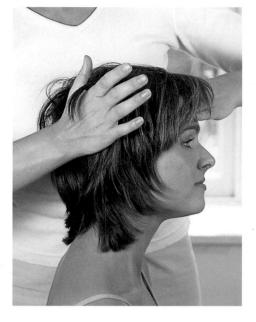

△ **2** Without stopping, use the heel of your right hand to rub briskly over the whole head as if you were buffing it up. Use firmer pressure at the base of the skull, repositioning yourself if necessary to get the heel of your hand under the occiput. Repeat three times. These strokes will increase circulation to the brain improving efficiency.

▽ **3** Standing behind your partner, slide both of your hands round to the side of the head. Spread your fingers wide and, with slow deliberate movements, make small circles on your partner's head, applying pressure with your fingertips. You should feel their scalp moving slightly. Using this "shampooing" action, work across the whole head. Repeat three times. This stroke releases the deeper layers of muscle that cover the head.

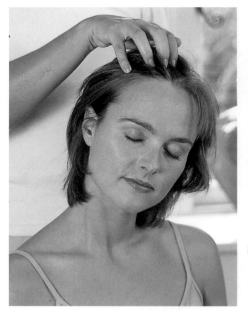

△ **4** Placing one hand at the top of your partner's forehead at the hairline, pull your fingers backwards through the hair in a strong raking movement. Let your other hand follow suit, building up a circular flow so that your partner doesn't have a sense of where one stroke begins and the other ends. Work over the whole head three times. Repeat this action with a slower, gentle ruffling movement through the hair, moving over the whole head three times.

▽ **5** Starting at the front hairline, use the whole of your hand to lightly stroke over your partner's head. Let one hand follow the other in a continuous movement and work down to the base of the skull. Work over the whole head a number of times. This stroking action is calming and soothing to the nervous system.

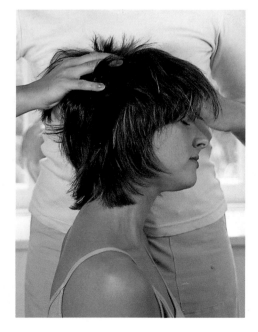

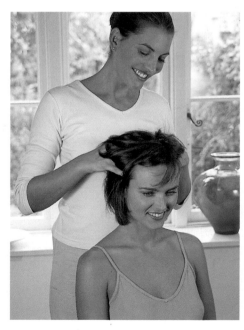

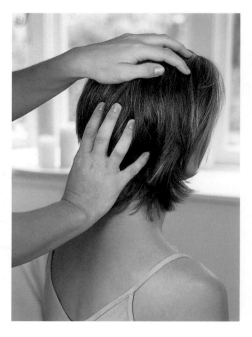

closing the sequence

The feeling of the ending is what will stay with
your partner after the massage has finished,
so make sure you don't end it too abruptly or
insensitively. To round off your treatment, slow
your actions down and take your time. Gentle
stroking or holding are ideal strokes to use, as
the hands gradually trail off the body. Make sure
your partner doesn't get up too quickly at the
end, but give them a glass of water and leave
them to sit for a while.

▷ **1** To close, trail your hands over the top of the
head and down the back using a brushing action as if
sweeping off cobwebs. Use one hand after the other
or both hands together, gradually coming to a stop.
Begin slowly and lightly. For a calming, reassuring end
finish in this way, and for an invigorating effect
increase to faster, firmer dynamic pressure .

▽ **2** Make sure that your partner is fully alert before
getting up, as massage works deeply, and it may take
them a while to come round.

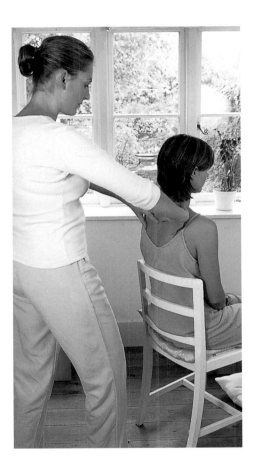

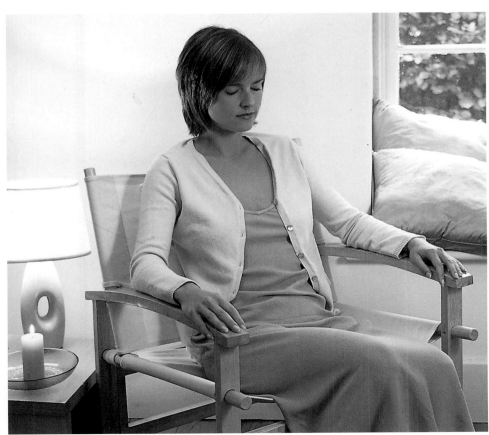

pressure points on the head

The head contains some key
pressure points. Massage strokes
that work well on these
acupressure points include friction
strokes, as in steps 1–3, and
tapotement or percussion and
pressure strokes, as in the basic
strokes section. If you wish to
apply direct pressure on the points
themselves, use the pads of your
fingers and gradually increase and
decrease the pressure as you come
off the points. Hold the pressure
for a few seconds only before
moving to the next points. Only
press as far as feels comfortable
for your partner.

Massage on the top of the head
relates to improvement in memory
and increased mental clarity. It also
helps to calm the spirit and clear
psychological conflicts. The points
at the base of the skull relate to
headaches, migraines and stiff
necks. The two points on the face
are connected with tension in the
shoulders and neck, and clearing
the lungs and chest of wheezing
and coughing.

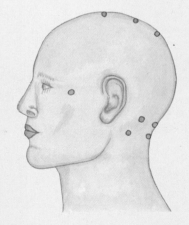

△ The location of the pressure points on
the face, head and base of the skull.

Head massage lying down

Sometimes you may prefer to give head massage with your partner lying down. This is ideal for when your partner has a headache, is very tired or has a backache from sitting all day. The advantage of lying down is that the neck and shoulder muscles no longer have to support the weight of the head and so have more chance to relax. The routine is similar to the sitting–up sequence except your partner is lying down.

preparation

The same preparation guidelines apply as with the standard sitting-up head massage routine, with one or two additional points to bear in mind. Before you begin, make sure that both you and your partner are comfortable. If your partner feels any discomfort, give their body some more support with cushions or towels beneath the knees or neck. If your partner wears contact lenses, they may want to remove them. Working from a kneeling or sitting position can be tiring, so have a cushion to sit or kneel on. Being uncomfortable during the massage is not only unpleasant for you but will also be communicated to your partner. Have a small bottle of lavender oil to hand in preparation for the face sequence.

▽ **Before you begin the massage make sure your partner is comfortable, and then ask them to lie still for a few moments with their hands resting gently on their stomach.**

head, neck and shoulders
If you are short of time, you can concentrate on massaging the head, neck and shoulders without having to work on the face.

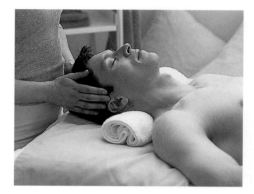

△ **1** Begin by gently placing your hands either side of your partner's head and hold it in this cradled position. Stay still for a few moments and attune your breathing with your partner's.

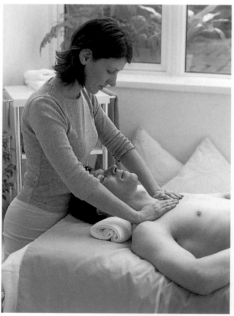

△ **2** Keeping contact with your hands, slide them down to the front of your partner's upper chest to just below the collarbone. The heels of your hands should be resting on the shoulders, with your hands forming a 'v' shape. Ask your partner to take a deep breath in; on the out-breath, press down with your hands, holding the pressure for as long as they breathe out. Repeat.

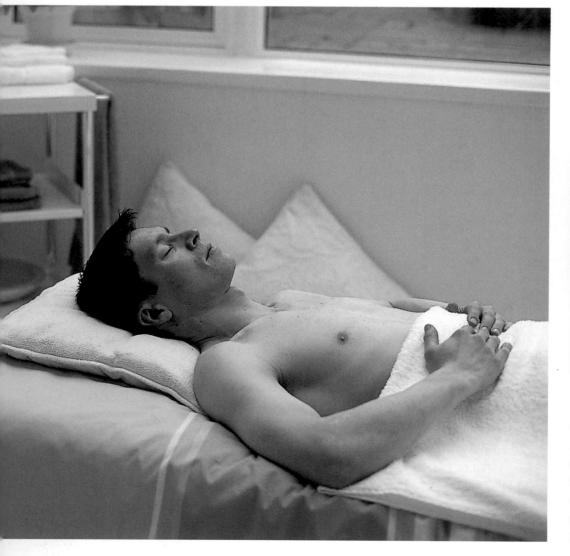

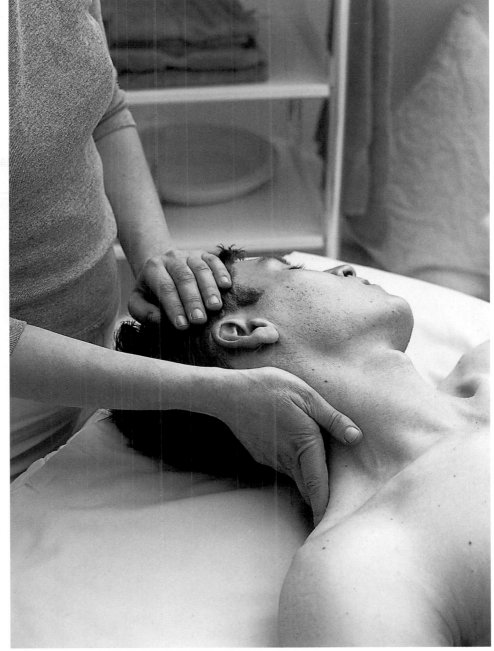

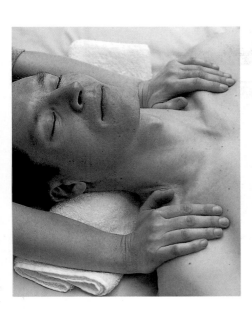

△ **3** Slowly draw your hands up to rest over the top of the shoulders. Listen to your partner's breathing, and as they breathe out push down on the shoulders in the direction of the feet. Repeat twice more.

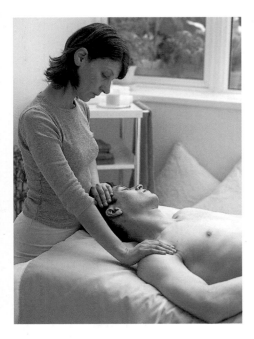

△ **4** Slide both your hands up to the sides of your partner's head and gently turn their head to one side. Keep one hand in position so it is cradling the head. Slide your other hand down the side of your partner's neck to the top of the shoulder. As your partner breathes out, push the shoulder down into the direction of the couch or floor. Repeat twice more.

△ **5** Place the palm of your hand at the base of the neck. Using the pads of your fingers, make circular strokes all the way up the side of the neck, being careful to avoid the windpipe area at the front. Then continue circling along the base of the skull, working from the middle towards the ear. Repeat twice. Then slide your hand to the side of your partner's head and turn the head back to a central position before repeating steps 4–5 on the other side.

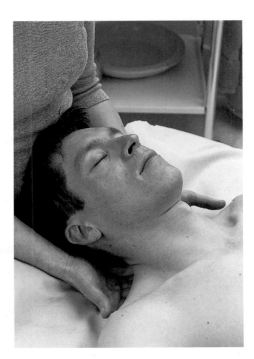

▷ **6** Slide your hands down the sides of the head to travel underneath the shoulders, with your fingertips at the base of the neck. Using the pads of your fingers, make circular strokes across the tops of the shoulders, and around the base of the neck. Continue circling underneath the shoulder blades, working into the muscles of the upper back. Discourage your partner from being "helpful" by lifting their spine.

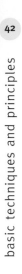

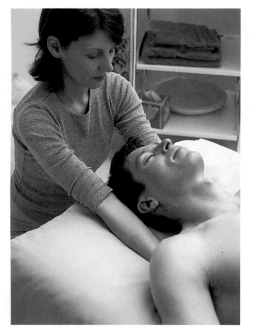

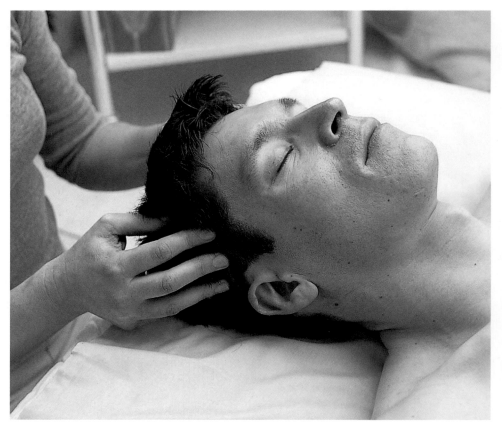

△ **7** Keep your hands underneath the back, palms facing up. Place your middle finger in the ridge that runs either side of the spine – it may be possible to reach as far down as the bottom of the shoulder blades. Ask your partner to take a deep breath in; on the out breath, slowly pull your hands up either side of the spine towards you. Continue the movement through to the top of the neck. Remove your hands and repeat twice more. This is a wonderful stretching stroke for the upper back and neck.

△ **9** Slide your hands to the back of the head. Starting at the back of the ears, use your fingertips to make circular strokes over your partner's scalp. You can either do this with both hands at once, or you may prefer to use one hand to work and the other to support the head. Pay particular attention to the area around the base of the skull, as a lot of tension accumulates here. As the tension loosens, try to feel the scalp moving underneath your fingertips. Work over the scalp three times.

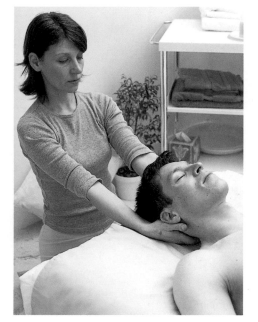

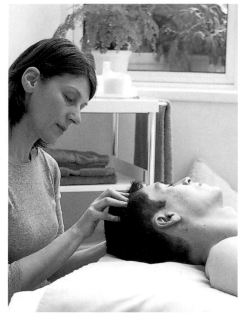

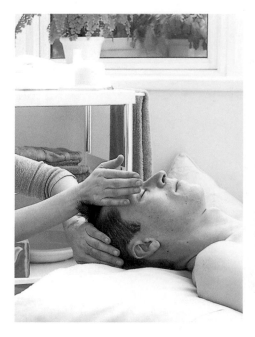

△ **8** Place both hands, one resting on top of the other, to cup underneath the neck. Slowly pull your hands up the length of the neck, gently lifting and stretching it towards you. Hold for a few seconds. Continue moving up and under the head, pulling your hands apart as you go until they come off the body at the top of the head. Repeat twice more.

△ **10** Position your right hand at the side of the head to support it and place the left at the base of the skull. Using the pads of your fingers, rub across the surface of the scalp in a zigzagging "windscreen wiper" movement. Work your way around the ears, increasing the depth of your massage to release tension. Cover the whole head three times.

△ **11** To finish on the head, stroke or comb through your partner's hair, using either your whole hand or just your fingers. Begin at the hairline and bring your hand down over the hair towards the back of the head. Let one hand lead and the other follow so it feels like a continuous movement. Cover the whole head three times, using lighter pressure to close.

working on the face

Ideally the full head massage sequence continues on the face, but you can perform this routine as a short facial sequence if you wish. When you have finished on the head, rub a drop of lavender oil between your palms to clear any residual smell from the scalp sweat glands and to provide a pleasant and calming aroma. The face contains many nerve endings that are very receptive to massage, accelerating the relaxation process.

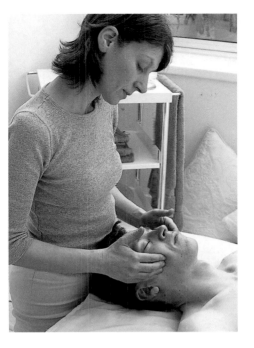

△ **2** This stroke involves circling movements over different areas of the face. Make sure that you cover each section three times and that you move smoothly from one area to the next. Using your fingertips, make small circular movements over the chin and above the upper lip. Continue with this circling action over the face, working well into the cheek and jaw area, which are both high tension spots, and using only feather-light pressure around the eye area.

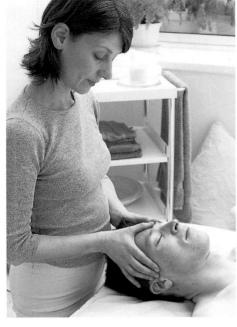

△ **4** Move your hands to the brow and let your thumbs meet together in the middle by the hairline. Using medium pressure, glide your thumbs in a straight line along the forehead and out towards the temples. Return your thumbs to the middle and work below the area just covered. Continue smoothing out the brow until the whole area is covered. Repeat twice more. This gentle but firm ironing out with the thumbs help to ease out worries and concerns registered in the lines of tension in the forehead.

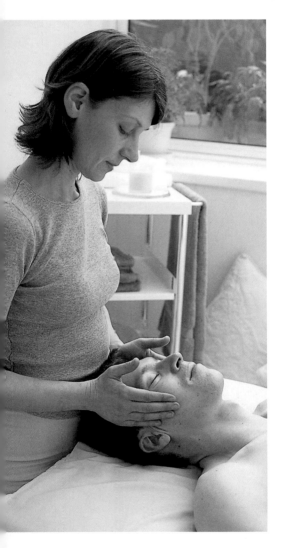

△ **1** Gently place both your hands on your partner's face, with your palms on either side of their chin. Lightly slide your hands up from the chin, stroking across the cheeks and up to the forehead. Repeat slowly several times, avoiding the delicate area around the eyes, and making your strokes a little firmer each time.

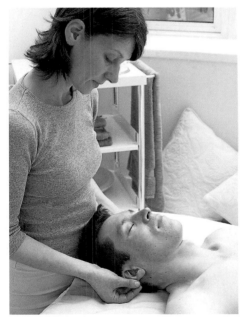

△ **3** Slide your fingers to your partner's ears. Starting at the top, use your thumbs and forefingers to lightly pinch or squeeze the ears' outer edges, working your way down to the base of the ear. End by pulling on each earlobe for a couple of seconds. Repeat three times and then cup your hands over the ears and hold for a few moments.

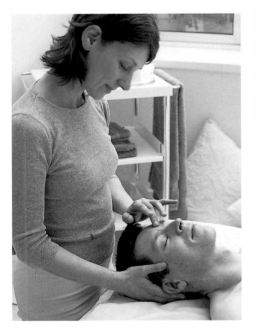

△ **5** To finish, place one finger in the "third eye" area, just above where the eyebrows would meet. Using light pressure, make small, slow circles over the surface of the skin, gradually increasing their size to take in more of the brow area. Make the circles smaller until your finger comes to a final resting place or stillness in the middle of the "third eye".

Self-massage

There are times when we could just do with a massage but there is no one around to oblige. Rather than give up, we can take a tip from other cultures, particularly those of the East, who have a longstanding tradition of self-massage. What we find is that head massage can be adapted into a self-treatment routine to suit ourselves in a wide variety of situations, as and when the need arises.

the shoulders and neck

You can follow the whole self-massage sequence, or if you have less time you can just work from the relevant section. It begins with the shoulders and neck. Make sure you are sitting comfortably with enough support for your spine, particularly if you feel tired. Many people find sitting cross-legged against a wall works well. Use cushions to give your back extra support if necessary.

▽ Prepare a nurturing space for yourself in which to self-massage, as this helps to create a healing atmosphere and to slow you down.

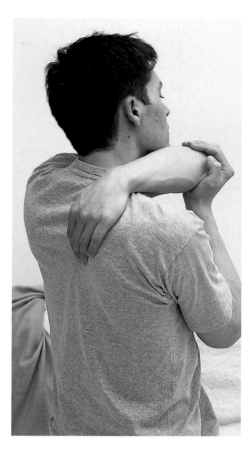

◁ **1** Take a deep breath in and out from your belly and place one hand on the opposite shoulder. This is your working hand. Lift your other hand and cup it over the elbow of your working hand for support and to provide leverage. Use your supporting hand to push the elbow up so that the working hand finishes as far down the upper back as is comfortable. Using the pads of your fingers make circular strokes, working your way upwards over the muscles that lie in between the shoulder blade and the spine. You can also massage around the line of the shoulder blade up to the top. Repeat twice more. Swap hands and repeat on the other side.

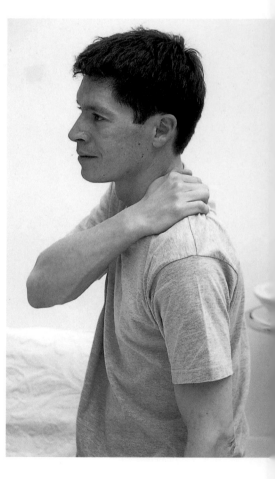

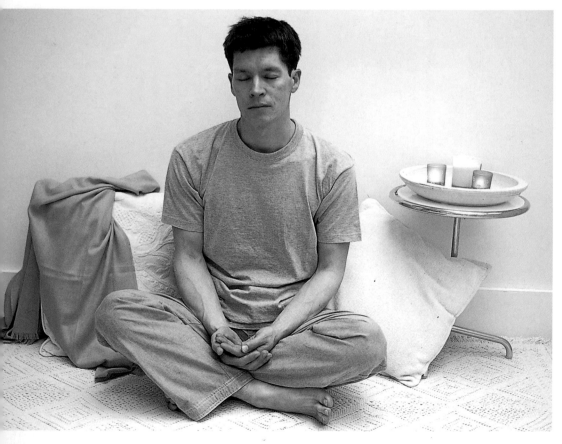

△ **2** Place your working hand near the base of your neck on the opposite shoulder. Using your whole hand, gently squeeze the muscle that starts here. Work your way along the top of the shoulder in this way, continuing down the upper arm to the elbow. Increase the intensity of pressure as you go if it is comfortable. Hold and release. Repeat three times. Swap hands and repeat on the other side.

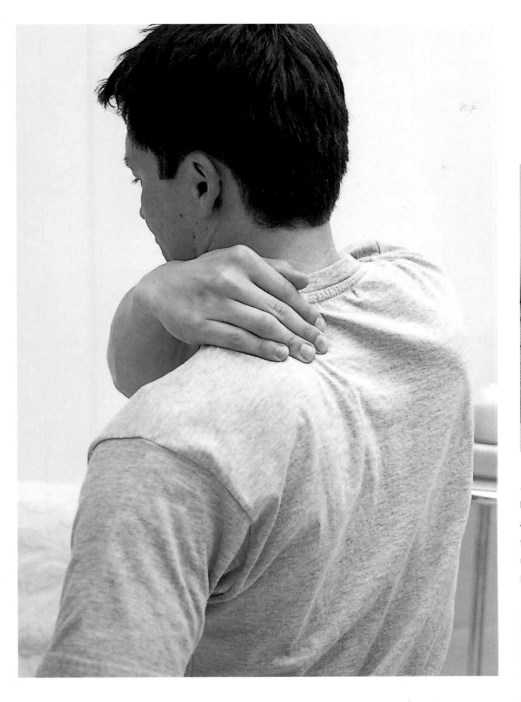

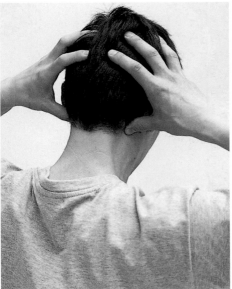

△ **5** Place one hand on your head and your working hand at the back of the neck. Tilt your head forwards a little. Starting at the top of the neck, use circular finger strokes to roll down the sides of the neck. Then use your whole hand to squeeze and pull down the back of the neck. Repeat three times and swap sides.

△ **3** Put your working hand at the base of the neck on the opposite shoulder, with your fingertips digging deep into the muscles. Using a circular action, work along the tops and backs of the shoulder muscles. Work as deeply as you can, concentrating on releasing areas of tension as you go. Work from the base of the neck out to the end of the shoulder. Repeat three times. Swap hands and repeat the process on the other side.

▷ **4** Place the thumb of your working hand in the hollow behind the collarbone. Using your other fingers, pinch and release along the tops of the shoulders. This might be quite painful if your muscles are tight, as it exerts pressure on the nerve endings, so remember to breathe out as you pinch. This stroke is very effective for releasing muscles that are taut or in spasm. Swap hands and repeat on the other side.

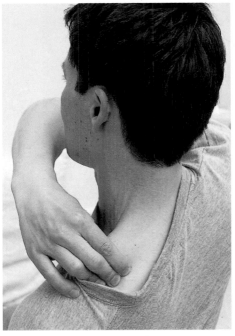

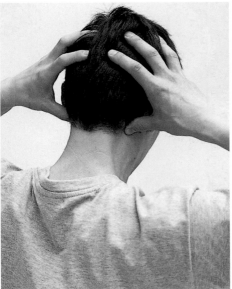

△ **6** Using both hands, clasp the back of your head and place your thumbs at the bony point just behind the ears. Work from here along the ridge of the skull, using thumb pressure and circular strokes from the middle outwards to the end to release tight muscle attachments. Repeat twice more.

the head

For the head part of the self-massage sequence, make sure you are sitting comfortably and adjust your position if necessary. Some people like to kneel or have their legs stretched out in front rather than sit cross-legged, which can be tiring. You can also do this sequence sitting down, with your elbows supported on a table.

▽ **1** Place your hands on your head and use the pads of your fingers to make circular strokes across your scalp. Work with medium pressure so that you feel the surface of the scalp move against the hard surface of the skull. You should feel this movement increase as you work. Cover the whole surface of the head three times, making sure that you work right down to the hairline.

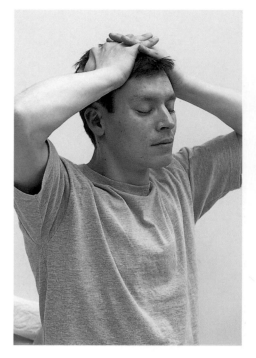

△ **2** With your hands on top of your head, interlock your fingers, press your palms into the sides of your head and lift them upwards. You should feel the scalp lift underneath your hands. Move to another part of the head and repeat, working in sections until the whole scalp is covered. If your hair is long enough, you can extend this lifting stroke by grabbing a fistful of hair with each hand and tugging it from side to side, keeping your knuckles close to the scalp.

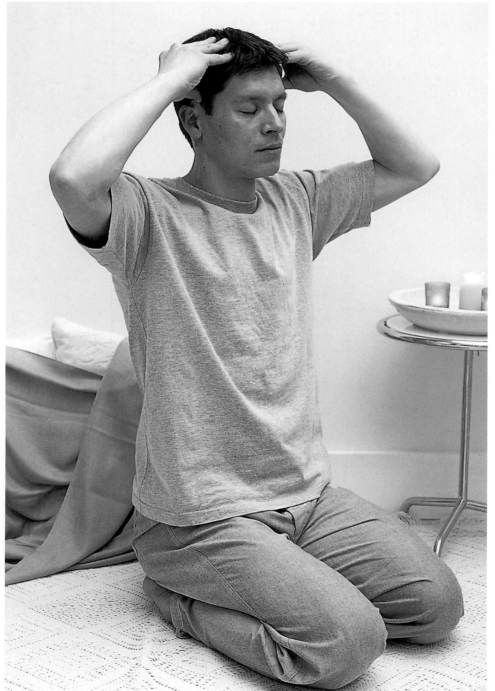

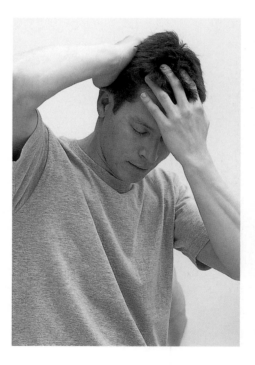

△ **3** Using both hands, use your fingers to rake through your hair and over your scalp. For a calming effect begin at the front of the head and work backwards to the nape of the neck. For an energising effect, begin at the nape of the neck and work forwards to the front. Repeat three times.

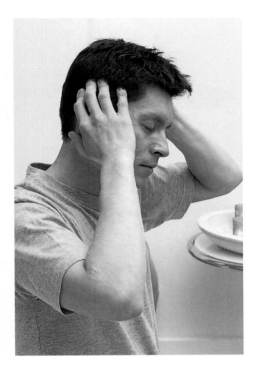

△ **4** Support your head with one hand on the side and put the other hand at the front of the ear by the hairline. Using the pads of your fingers, rub vigorously backwards and forwards in a friction stroke, applying medium pressure. Pay particular attention to releasing the muscle band that runs around and across the top of the ear. Massage the whole head using this stroke three times, working in a fast rhythmical way and changing hands when necessary.

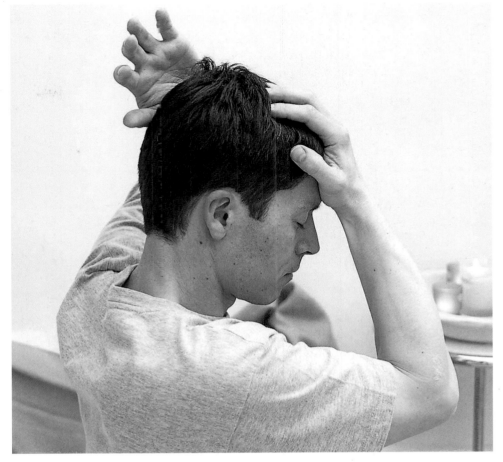

△ **6** Use one hand to support your head at the front. Put your other hand at the base of the skull in the middle and use the heel of your hand in a zigzagging motion to rub up and over the back of the head until one side is completely covered. Change hands and repeat on the other side.

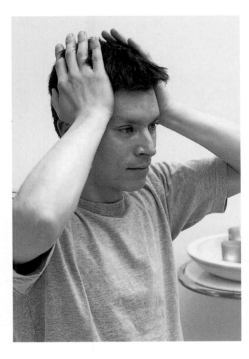

△ **5** Place the heels of both hands on your temples. Press in slightly and make circular actions with your hands. Keep your movements slow and work in a clockwise and then an anti-clockwise direction. Adjust pressure so that it is comfortable to receive. Repeat five times in each direction.

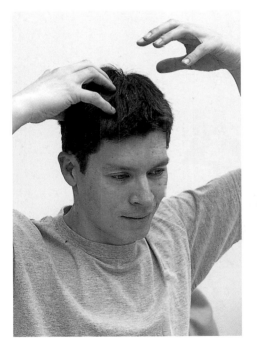

△ **7** Place the tips of your fingers on top of your head and begin to tap lightly all over the surface of the head, building up a smooth rhythm as you work. Keep your fingers soft so that your touch is light and your fingers spring off the surface of the head. Work over the whole head three times.

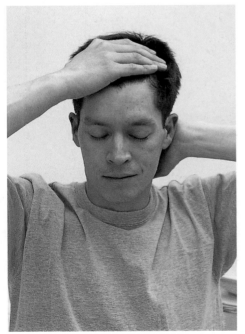

△ **8** Make long stroking movements working from the front of the head to the nape of the neck. As one hand comes off the head, let the other come down so that one stroke flows seamlessly into another. Cover the whole head a few times, gradually slowing down until you finally come to a stop.

the face

Most of us are unaware of how much tension we store in our faces, particularly around the jaw area. The tightness it registers leaves us looking tired and strained. Using self-massage on your face is soothing and relaxing, especially at the end of a long and stressful day, and will help restore a fresher look to your face. This sequence can be done as a facial massage in its own right. Again make sure you are sitting comfortably with your back well supported.

▽ **1** Place your thumbs just under your chin with the pads of your fingers resting on top. Now, pressing your thumb and fingers together, pinch your way along the whole of the lower jaw line. As you get to the outer edge of the jaw, you can increase the pressure as a lot of tension is usually held here. Work along the whole area three times. There are a lot of lymph nodes along the jaw line and this action stimulates their function to eliminate toxins from the body. Extend this stroke by making circular strokes with your fingers over the chin and lower jaw area.

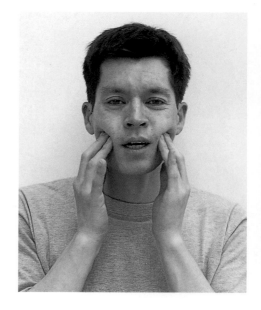

△ **2** Using the pads of your fingers, make circular strokes across the whole of your face. Begin at the bottom by the jaw line and work upwards using light pressure. To avoid stretching the skin, only use the pressure on the upward movements and be especially careful with the delicate area around the eyes. Cover the surface of your face three times. Around the jaw area and cheeks you can make your circling action slower and deeper, working deeply into the jaw socket itself to release tension.

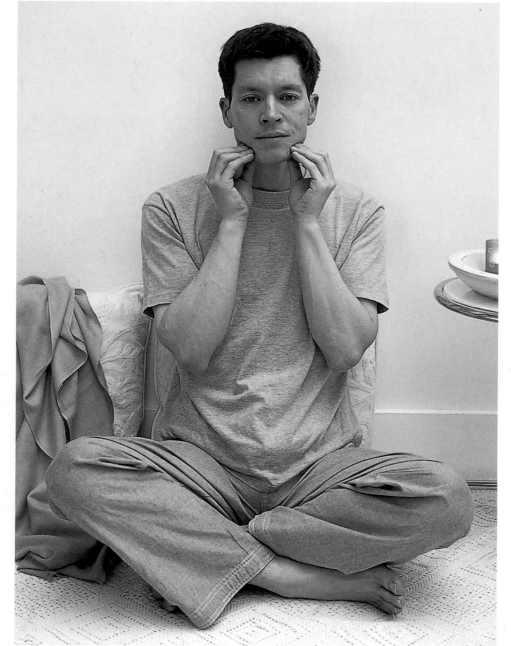

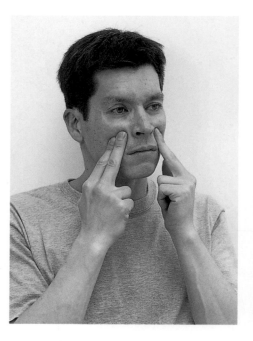

△ **3** Place your first two fingers on the underside of your cheeks, near the hollow at the base of your nose. Press in gently against the bone, hold and release. Move along the cheekbone with this action until you get to the hinge by the jawbone, then work your way back to the middle of the face. Repeat this movement three times. Any tender spots can indicate areas of sinus congestion, which may be helped by this particular massage action.

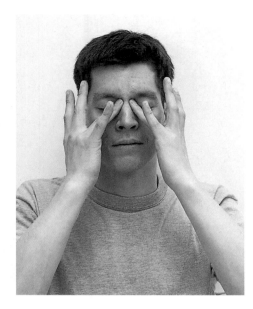

△ **4** Close your eyes and put the pads of your ring fingers at the inner edge of your eyebrows by the bridge of the nose. Gently but firmly press inwards and upwards, hold for a few seconds and then release. Repeat a few more times if the area feels tender, which indicates congestion. Continue with this pressure stroke, working out along the lower edge of the eyebrow and back underneath the eye, tracing the bony rim of the eye. Complete three full circles in this way.

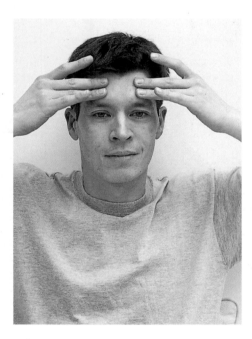

△ **5** Place your middle fingers on your forehead so that they face tip to tip in the middle of your lower brow. Slowly draw your fingers apart across the brow towards the hairline. Move your fingers a little higher up the forehead and repeat. Continue to work up the brow in sections, smoothing out lines of worry and tension as you go. Cover the whole area three times. To draw to a close, use your fingers to trace increasingly light circles around the "third eye" area.

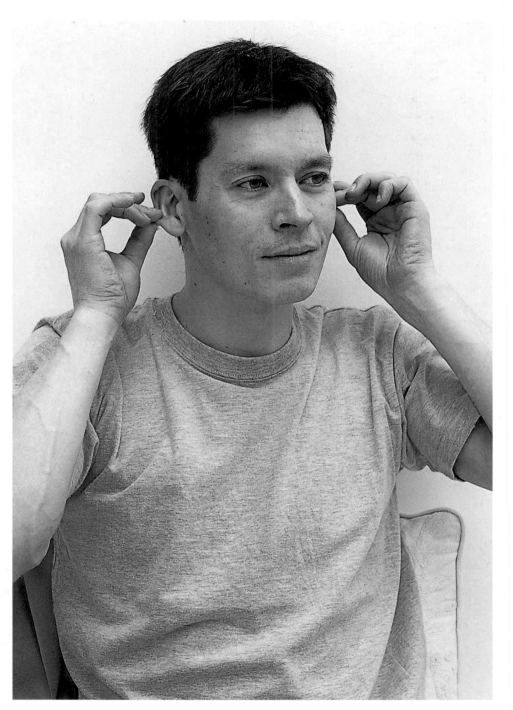

△ **6** With thumb and fingertips at the bottom of both earlobes, gently squeeze and roll along the outer edge of the ears, working up to the top. At the top, continue squeezing and rolling down the inner edge of the ears, back to where you began. Repeat this movement twice, then gently pull down on the earlobes to release them. Next place your palms over your ears and rub over the area, exerting a comfortable pressure. Do this a number of times. You can rub quite briskly till your ears are quite warm for a stimulating effect. This ear massage action will have an energizing result and will help relieve pain being experienced elsewhere in the body, as the ears contain correspondences to the whole system. The stimulating effect will activate the body's energy channels (meridians). To finish the massage sequence, gently place your palms against your ears for a few moments and slowly release.

Five-minute fixes

When you don't have enough time for a complete self-massage sequence, there are some quick-fix routines that can be done at home or at work. They will give you an energy boost, keep your body loose and help improve posture. The first five-minute routine is based on shiatsu-style massage and works on energy channels; the second sequence focuses on neck care and includes a sequence of movements that can be done at any time during the day.

energy channels booster

The following massage routine is energizing and invigorating. It works by activating the energy channels (meridians) that run throughout the body through the use of tapping and pummelling movements. It "wakes up" the whole body and is therefore ideal for first thing in the morning or if you need recharging in the middle of the day. The energizing, pummelling action of your knuckles also has a stimulating effect on some of the muscles, increasing peripheral circulation and loosening tension through its vibrations.

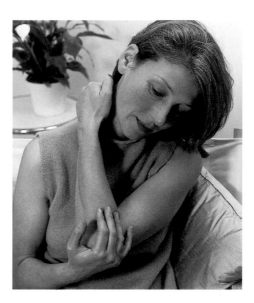

△ **1** Sit with your shoes off. Spread out your toes and plant your feet firmly on the ground. Cup your left elbow in the palm of your right hand and use your left knuckles to tap the right side of the body. Tap down the side of the neck and continue over the top of the shoulder and down into the upper back. Work as far down the back as you can, using your hand on your elbow for leverage. Repeat on the other side.

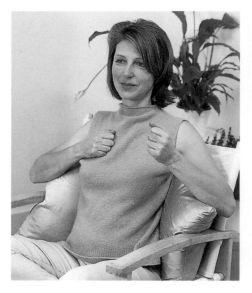

△ **3** Now use the same tapping stroke on your chest. Sit back in the chair and, keeping your wrists soft, tap across the upper chest. Work from the middle of your chest outwards towards the shoulder. This is a very invigorating and sometimes quite amusing movement. Repeat three times.

trapezius muscles

Under stress these muscles tighten and can pull the muscles around the neck and on the attachments to the skull, resulting in headaches, stiffness, and impaired breathing. Stretching helps reduce and prevent this build up of tension.

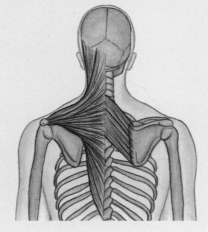

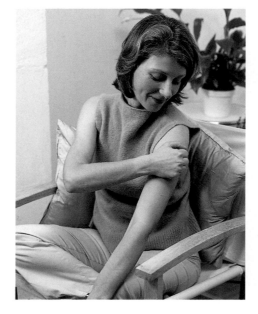

△ **2** Continue tapping down the outside of your arm to your hand. Then tap up on the inside all the way up to the armpit, over the shoulder joint and then back down the outside of the arm once more. Repeat three times, then swap hands and do the other arm.

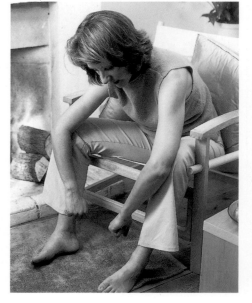

△ **4** Place your feet slightly apart on the ground, and pummel down the outside of both legs at the same time. Repeat this action three times. Finish by pummelling up the inside of both legs. Repeat three times. Slowly sit up and take a deep breath to finish.

essential neck care

Weaknesses, tension and imbalances in the neck are helped and can even be corrected by exercise. These gentle movements will loosen up and strengthen the neck, giving greater freedom of movement and reducing the risk of strain or injury. They only take a few minutes and are effective for stretching out the muscles and connective tissue and energizing the body. They can also help improve posture. It is important to keep breathing during exercises to encourage the flow of oxygen to the muscles and assist the releasing process.

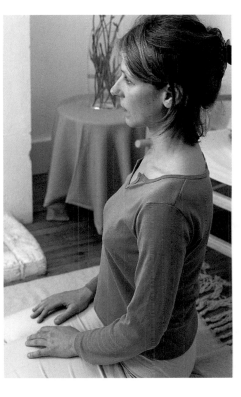

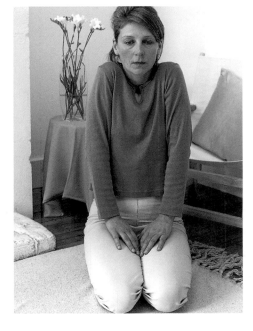

▽ A poor posture profile, such as a curved back, slumped shoulders and a head that juts forwards is commonplace. Stretching, exercises and massage help reverse the trend and prevent this posture becoming a long term hump that is set and irreversible in later years.

To improve your posture, kneel on the floor, take a deep breath in, and on the out breath drop your shoulders. Imagine your head is attached to a cord tied to the ceiling. Every time you breathe out imagine the cord pulling your head up, and your spine lengthening and straightening.

△ **1** Take a deep breath in and slowly begin to lift your shoulders up and back as far as they will comfortably go. On the out breath, slowly release, beginning the upward movement again on the next in breath. As your shoulder blades come down, imagine them meeting together in the middle of your back. Shoulder shrugs help to release tension in the large muscles of the upper back that pull on the neck.

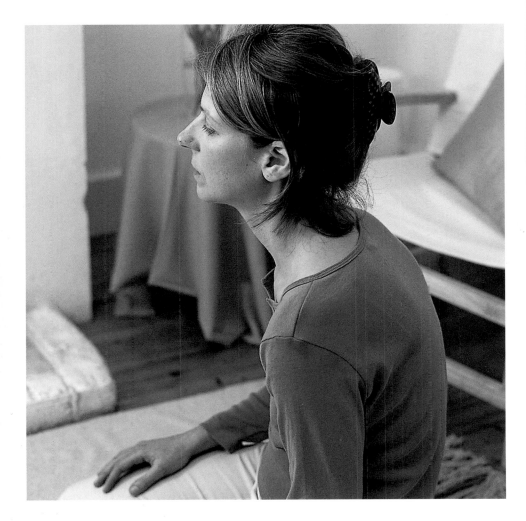

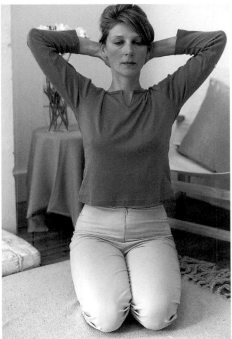

△ **2** Centre your head and tuck your chin in. Tuck your hands behind your head, push your head against them and hold for 3–5 seconds. Repeat 10–20 times. Then place one hand on the side of your head. Tuck your chin in, push your head against your hand and hold for 3–5 seconds. Repeat 10–20 times. Swap hands and repeat on the other side. These movements help to strengthen the neck muscles.

Energy work

There is more to the body than meets the eye. As you approach another person, they may be able to sense your presence before you touch them. That is because you have entered their "energy field" or aura, the invisible vibrations that radiate from our bodies. The stronger and healthier we are, the bigger and more expansive our aura; when we are tired or sick, this field is smaller and closer to the body. The chakra system is part of this energy field and some understanding of it is useful in head massage. Although you may not be able to see it, you will be affecting the way it functions through your touch.

health and the chakras

The chakras represent energy points in the body. The word *chakra* means "wheel" in Sanskrit, indicating that the chakras are like

▽ Spiritual awareness is part of Eastern culture and in India it is commonplace to see the "third eye" marked by wearing a bindi.

spinning vortexes, receiving energy from the universe and transforming it to be utilized by the body. In energy-based medicine, the first signs of ill health are believed to show up as blockages or disturbances in the chakras. If these imbalances are not sorted out then the issue will eventually show up as a physical problem. Keeping the chakras working effectively is important for good health.

the chakra system

There are seven major chakras, each having its own characteristics and correspondences. They run up the body from the base of the spine to the top of the head and can be located on the front and back of the body. Each chakra is associated with different organs and systems of the body and with a different colour, although there are some variations according to which chakra system you are using. In head massage we are concerned with the four higher chakras: the heart, throat, "third eye" and crown.

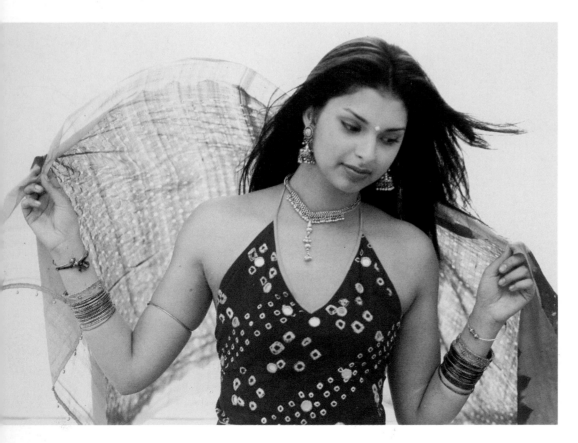

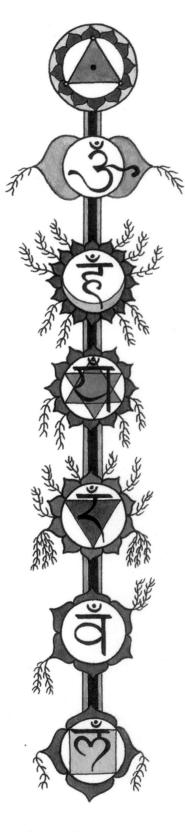

△ The seven major chakras are energy centres for accessing and distributing *chi* or *prana* or life force around the body through the system of meridian channels.

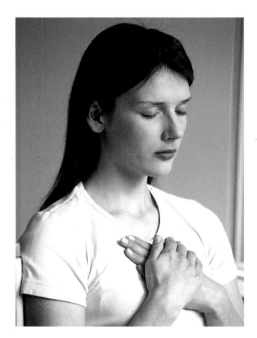

△ Resting your hands over your heart centre and breathing into the hold will help you feel your own heart energy through which love and healing forces flow.

upper body chakras

Roughly halfway up the spine, the heart chakra corresponds to unconditional love, compassion, empathy and friendship. Physically it relates to the thymus, heart, lungs, bronchial tubes, upper back and the arms. It is associated with pink and green and is the home of the soul. As you work on the upper back you will be in its sphere. The physical release points for the heart chakra are in the shoulders, the intercostal muscles of the ribs, the upper arms, under the chin and at the base of the skull.

The throat chakra is located at the base of the neck where it connects to the shoulders. It corresponds to turquoise or sky blue and is concerned with all forms of communication and self-expression. It speaks the words of your soul. Unexpressed feelings may show up as a blockage in this chakra and lead to throat problems. In the body it relates to the thyroid, ear, nose and throat, the neck and teeth. Its physical release points are in the neck, shoulders, fingers and toes.

The "third eye" chakra is located in the middle of the forehead or the brow. In India this spot is often marked with a bindi, sandalwood paste, or kohl. Its energy release points are in the eyes, temples, forehead and at the base of the skull. It corresponds to indigo or royal blue and is concerned with the development and deepening of intuition and soul knowledge. It regulates the energies of the pituitary and nervous systems, as well as the brain, head, eyes and face.

The crown chakra is located at the top of the head. Its energy release points are in the head, hands and feet. It is associated with purple or violet and is concerned with higher consciousness and spirituality.

working with the chakras

As you massage, you can become aware of these energy centres, especially when working near the areas of the body where they reside. At the end of a treatment, when your partner is still, you could experiment by using "holds" over one or two chakras. To do this, place one hand gently over the other and let them rest lightly over a chakra spot for a few moments. Follow your intuition when choosing each spot. For instance, if you sense your partner needs comfort and reassurance, then you may feel drawn to the heart chakra in the middle of the upper back. Or if your partner has communication issues, then a gentle holding on the throat chakra at the back of the neck may be the spot. As you "hold" imagine healing energy flowing from your heart chakra down your arms and out of your hands in to your partner, and intend that it goes where it is most needed.

When you have finished, take your hands away slowly and carefully. See if you can feel your partner's energy field and notice the point at which your hands finally leave it. It is likely that after a treatment their energy field will have expanded, as the chakras have become more balanced and their energies are flowing more efficiently.

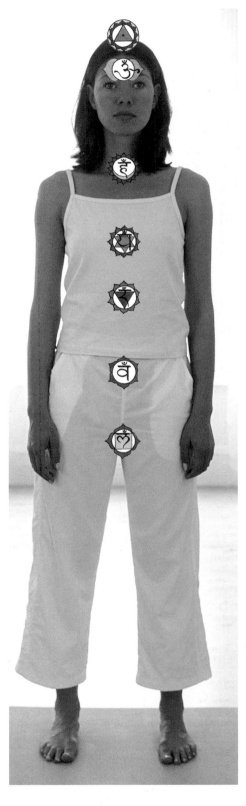

△ The chakras are located in key areas and these energies nourish, and have correspondences with, the physical and emotional dimensions of the whole person.

Relieving stress at work

Technological advances have revolutionized our working patterns. Many of these changes are associated with computers and an increase in sedentary jobs, which in turn is leading to a build-up of tension in the body and an increase in emotional stress. This is because our bodies are designed for movement, and our muscular structure functions most effectively when it is used in a whole, active and dynamic way. Increasingly this is not the case. We move in limited ways and hold our bodies in relatively static positions for extended periods of time. This is creating a range of common problems. It is in this context that massage becomes such a valuable tool for relieving stress in the workplace.

work stress

A typical office worker is likely to hold their back, neck, shoulders, arms and eyes in static positions for long periods of time. This causes the muscles to "freeze" into an almost permanent state of tension, in which they no longer work efficiently. The flow of nutrients, oxygen and blood supply is restricted, reducing the efficient circulation of blood to the brain and throughout the body. This leads to tiredness and irritability, as well as poor concentration and difficulties with decision-making. If the muscles are not released through movement or manipulation, they contract and toxins build up in the muscle tissue. This reduces mobility and causes all manner of aches and pains, while specific work-related conditions, such as repetitive strain injury (RSI) and carpal tunnel syndrome, are becoming increasingly common.

On top of the physical stress, many people experience psychological stress at work, which usually makes the physical discomfort worse. Time limits, dealing with frustration or feeling pressurized to perform can all literally become "a pain in the neck" if emotional pressures are not discharged at some point.

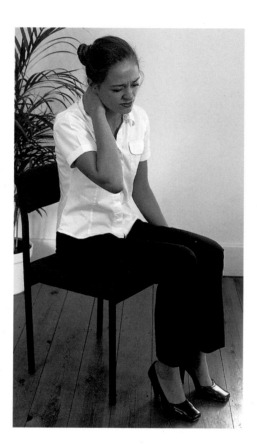

△ Sitting down working at a desk or computer for long periods of time often causes tension and pain in the neck and shoulders.

self-help measures

Current thinking says that for every hour that you spend working at a computer screen, you should take a ten-minute break. During this time you should do something active to help discharge physical tension. This could include self-massage, stretch and release exercises or massage with a co-worker. Done regularly, such measures will help discharge tension, particularly from the upper body. They will also help to keep body and mind relaxed and alert during the whole working day.

releasing neck tension

With one hand, grab a handful of flesh from the back of your neck. Squeeze it as hard as feels comfortable and hold the pressure, slowly nodding your head up and down at the same time. Mentally say the word "yes" to yourself as you do this. Keep breathing as you repeat this movement a couple of times. Swap hands, and this time shake your head from side to side, mentally saying "no" inside your head.

neck and shoulder stretch

This stretch helps to release tight neck and shoulder muscles and can be done standing or sitting. Lift one arm and bend it so that your hand is facing palm down on your upper back. Take your other arm and bend it so that your hand reaches up your back with the palm facing outwards. Move both hands towards each other so that the fingers meet and clasp together. If the hands do not reach one another, then rest them as close together as possible. Hold for 15 seconds, maintaining a steady breathing rhythm. Change hands and repeat the stretch on the other side, again holding it for 15 seconds while breathing steadily.

▽ Taking regular breaks to release taut neck muscles with self-massage contributes greatly to preventing the gradual build up of chronic tension.

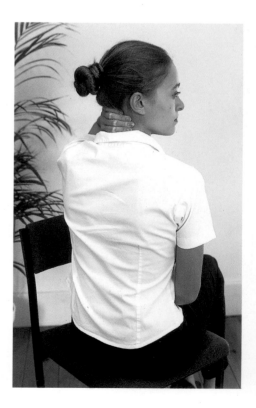

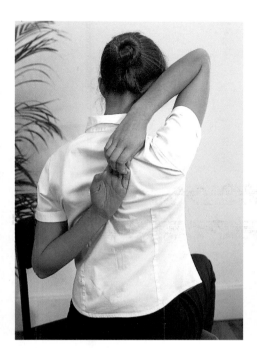

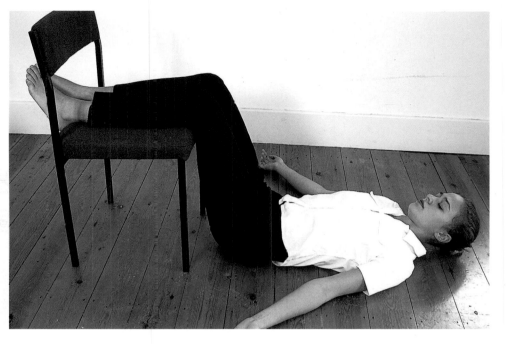

△ Stretching breaks help release and promote deeper breathing, which oxygenates the body and brain, increasing brain functioning.

resting the eyes

Our eye muscles get surprisingly tired from focusing for long periods on a fixed plane of vision, such as a computer screen. This simple palming exercise will give your eyes a rest and help to release taut eye muscles. Vigorously rub your hands together so that they become warm and energized, then place them over your eyes, your fingers

▽ It is important to rest your eyes following periods of concentrated work as this helps to prevent strain and stress, which contribute to headaches and impaired vision.

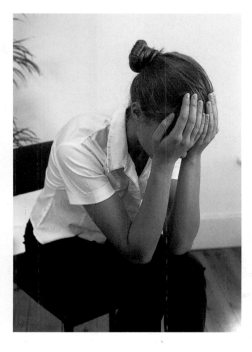

resting on your forehead. Close your eyes. Hold for a few minutes while your eyes rest in the darkness of your hands. Use the time to tune in to your breathing and focus on letting go of tension as you breathe out.

back, neck and shoulder release

The following exercise should help release tension in the upper back, neck and shoulders. It encourages the effective flow of blood back to the head and brain and is ideal after an extended period of deskwork, such as at lunchtime. If you cannot do it at your own desk, you may be able to find another suitable place such as an unused conference or meeting room.

Sit on the floor at right angles to a chair. Then swivel around so that you are facing the chair and put the lower half of your legs up. Your feet and calves should be resting flat on the chair and your knees should be bent at right angles with the floor. Let your arms fall out to the sides with palms facing upwards. Wriggle your back and adjust your position so that your spine is as flat as possible on the floor. It is best if you can close your eyes and rest in this position for at least five minutes.

Gently breathe in and out and use your imagination to visualize the fresh flow of oxygen, blood and nutrients flowing up through your back, shoulders, neck and head to your brain and then down again. This will help to replenish and recharge your upper body and head.

△ Lying down so that your spine can be supported by the ground gives it a chance to decompress and rehydrate, leaving you feeling refreshed and alert.

co-worker massage

Massage between work colleagues can create a much happier atmosphere. This is a very quick and easy routine. Sit your partner in front of you and gently rest your forearms on their shoulders. Ask them to take a deep breath in and on the out breath, press down on their shoulders. Then use the whole of your hands to rub briskly over their shoulders and upper back.

▽ Making co-worker massage part of your work culture makes a noticeable difference in terms of increased creativity and efficiency.

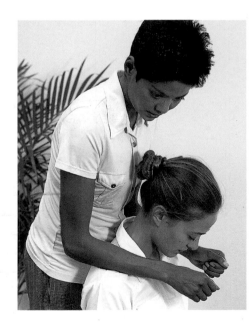

End of the day de-stresser

Being able to relax and leave work behind is essential if we are to make the most of our time off. Yet with the day's work over, many people find that switching off is not so simple and have trouble letting go of stress and tension. Head massage is a fantastic tool for de-stressing after a long day, whether you've been out at work or involved in childcare at home. Many people find it much more effective than other quick-fix solutions, such as drinking alcohol, as its benefits are longer lasting and it has no harmful side effects. An end of the day de-stress routine can be done with a partner or by yourself – even if you feel too tired to bother, it's usually well worth the effort.

partner shoulder massage

Massage with your partner gives both of you the opportunity to relax and to re-connect after being in different worlds all day. It can form part of winding down and spending quality time together, and after just a few minutes of massaging the shoulders the cares and tensions of the day will start to fade as your muscles begin to unwind.

▽ **1** Briskly rub the palm of your hand over your partner's shoulders and upper back, and use fingers and thumbs to massage knots and tensions away.

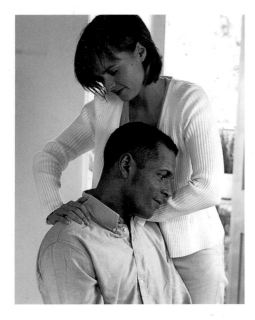

after work de-stresser

After you have been sitting at work all day, the following sequence is specifically designed to target the areas of stress in the body. It is done lying down to give your muscles and spine a chance to decompress. Make sure that you have a firm, comfortable surface to lie on, plus cushions for support and a blanket for keeping warm. Turn the lights down low and make sure the phone is off the hook.

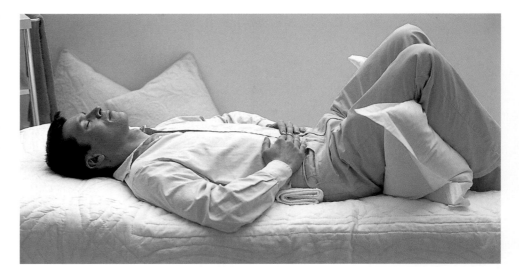

△ **1** Begin by lying flat on your back. Bending your knees is helpful, as it gives the lower back extra support and helps the spine to lengthen and straighten. You could also place a large cushion underneath your knees as a bolster. Place your hands on your belly, close your eyes and take a few deep breaths in and out of your belly. As you breathe in, you should feel your hands lift up slightly and as you breathe out feel your belly contract and your hands come back in. Do this a few times.

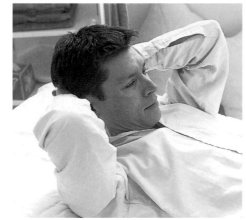

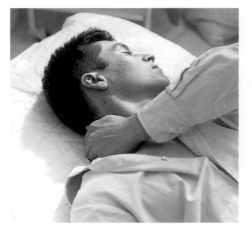

△ **2** Clasp your hands together behind your head. As you breathe slowly out, lift your head up with them. The hands should lead with the head following. Do this slowly, imagining each vertebra lifting one at a time as you rise. When the neck is comfortably stretched, hold for a few moments and release slowly and smoothly, vertebra by vertebra. Repeat twice.

△ **3** Turn your head to the left and place your left hand on the right side of your neck. Using the fleshy pad of your hand (by the base of the thumb), make small circles, working down the neck and continuing across the top of the shoulders. Increase the size of the circles as you go. Repeat three times and then do the same on the other side.

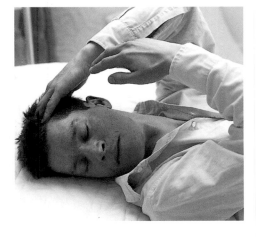

△ **6** With your left hand on your right shoulder, place your thumb in the hollow behind the collarbone and the remaining fingers over the top of the shoulder. Squeeze your thumb and fingers together, and on the out breath pinch this muscle and hold for as long as you can. Release and repeat at intervals along both shoulders till you have pinched both three times.

△ **8** Run your fingers across your scalp as if you were combing and lifting your hair away from your head. Flick your fingers away as they come off the ends of the hair. You can either do this stroke softly and slowly for a relaxing effect, or firmer and faster for an energizing clearing effect. Work over the whole of your head three times.

△ **4** Move your head back to the left and press your right thumb into the bony ridge behind the ear. Press, hold and release. Continue working in this way along the edge of the skull towards the middle. Aim for comfortable pressure, repeat twice and swap sides.

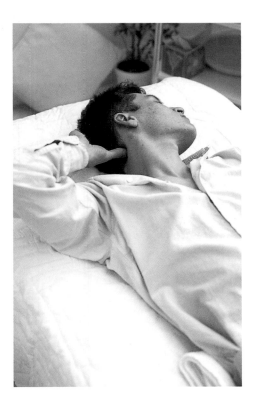

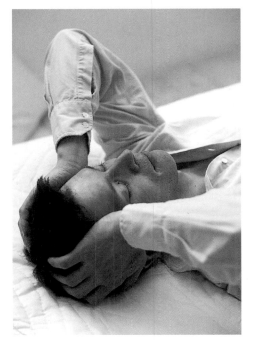

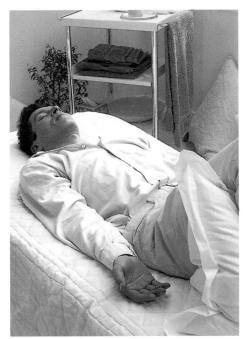

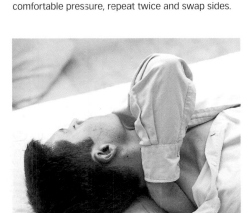

△ **5** With your head on the left, hook your left hand over your right shoulder, resting the heel on top of the shoulder with the fingers pointing down the back. Dig your fingers into the muscle, grab some flesh and drag it up until your fingers slide over your shoulder. Continue finding tight spots along both shoulders. Repeat three times on both sides.

△ **7** Place the heels of your hands or your temples and, using medium to firm pressure, press while simultaneously making circles. Make at least six big slow circles and work into areas of tension. If you wish, you can extend this circling act on to include the whole head and scalp, using the heel of your hands or your fingers.

△ **9** To finish, take a deep breath in and out from your belly as in the beginning. Rest for a few moments, covering yourself with a blanket, if you wish. Imagine stale energy and stress leaving your body as you breathe out, and fresh energy revitalizing your body and mind as you breathe in. When you are ready, roll on to one side and get up slowly.

Relieving tension from driving

Driving is an integral part of a modern sedentary lifestyle. We use our cars to make short journeys around town as well as for longer trips and we spend a lot of time behind the steering wheel. For most of us, our cars are indispensable, yet driving can also create stress and tension in the body. To minimize this we can cultivate some good driving habits. These include improving and adjusting our driving posture, taking breaks during long journeys and using some stretching and self-massage treatments to ease out tense muscles.

improving posture

How you sit at the wheel is a key to body tension. Bad habits include craning your neck to peer over the driving wheel or overextending your back by leaning too far backwards. The body's muscles then become tired and stressed, leading to aches and pains. If the back's lumbar region is not supported, it can have a tendency to sag and slump. This pulls on the muscles and puts a strain on the rest of the spine.

▽ **Driving in poor conditions, a hurry or heavy traffic can all contribute to poor posture and can have the effect of making it worse.**

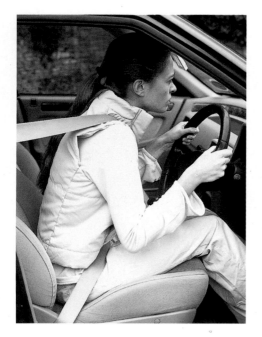

Good posture supports the body's musculature and helps keep its energies flowing. Make sure that you sit up straight and that your seat supports you. You can use cushions to adjust your position, or buy the special back supports now available. Have enough headroom between your head and the roof of the car, otherwise you may slouch to fit yourself into the available space. Adjust all the mirrors so you can see them without straining. Hold the middle of the steering wheel, keeping your arms relaxed. Don't twist your feet. They should be in line with your legs and facing forwards.

Sitting for prolonged periods in the same position impairs circulation and causes the body to stiffen up. This can lead to aches and pains in your neck and back, arms and wrists, or legs and ankles. It can also result in eyestrain and headaches, as well as lower levels of mental alertness.

To avoid freezing in the same position, make little postural adjustments as you drive. For instance, you can wriggle yourself further back into your seat, or if you are stuck in traffic, try relaxing your shoulders by lifting and releasing them. As you drive check periodically that your jaw is relaxed, your shoulders stay soft and that you are breathing from your abdomen.

▽ **Sitting in an upright position with a supported back can help make driving safer and minimizes the build-up of tension.**

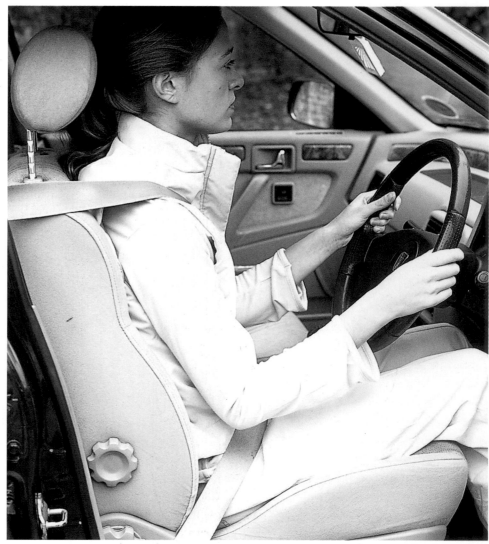

body stretches

On long journeys it is very important to take regular breaks to have some fresh air and a chance to stretch. This will help to release tension, improve circulation and restore concentration, making you a more relaxed and effective driver. Research now shows that taking regular massage and stretch breaks while driving has a beneficial effect on improving driver concentration and on reducing the number of road accidents. It has been shown to be much more effective than coffee breaks.

These stretches and massages are easy to do wherever you take a break from driving. Do each one a number of times. The stretches mobilize the spine, lower back, arms and shoulders.

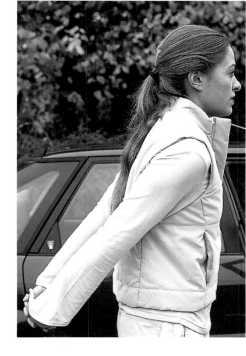

△ **2** Clasp your hands together behind your back. As you breathe out, bring them up slowly as far as possible. Hold and release slowly as you breathe in. Release your arms and let them drop down. Repeat at least three more times. This helps relieve tightness in the shoulders and between the shoulder blades.

self-massage tension relievers

You can also try this quick-fix self-massage during a driving break or when you get home. It will help to ease out tension in the head, neck, and shoulder areas.

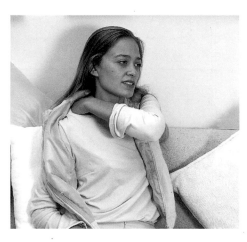

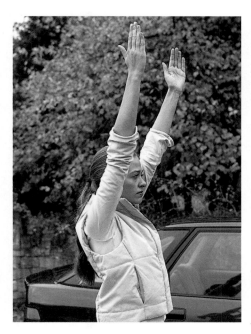

△ **1** Stand with your feet together and facing forwards. Breathe in and stretch your arms up above your head, lengthening up through your spine. On the out breath, bend your knees, tuck your chin in and roll your spine down, vertebra by vertebra, slowly bending forwards as far as is comfortable. Bring your arms down as you do this movement and let them swing gently backwards and forwards. On an in breath, bring your arms forwards and lengthen up through your body to come up to standing.

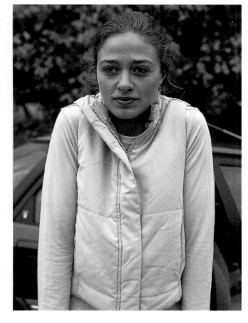

△ **3** Take a deep breath in and slowly begin to lift your shoulders up as far as they will comfortably go. Hold them up tightly as near your ears as possible. As you breathe out, let your shoulders drop abruptly in a release. You can extend this stretch by lifting and rolling your shoulders forwards as slowly as possible. Then change directions so that you roll your shoulders backwards. It can help if you try to imagine your shoulder blades meeting together in the middle of your back as you circle them.

△ **1** Sit with your back well supported and place one hand over the opposite shoulder. Make small circular strokes across the shoulder using your fingertips. Work your way down into the upper back and along the edge of your shoulder blade as far down as you can. As your hand returns up your back, massage the muscles between your shoulder blade and spine.

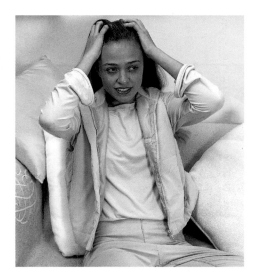

△ **2** Using your fingertips, rub back and forth across the top of your shoulder, following the muscles up into the side of your neck. Continue the movement up to your head, working around the whole head with this rubbing motion.

Asthma management

Asthma is a breathing disorder that affects one in seven of the population. It can occur at any age and involves inflammation of the bronchial tubes, excess mucus production and the contraction of muscles in the chest area. This narrowing of the air passages restricts the flow of oxygen and leads to breathing difficulties. These can range from a mild tightening in the chest to restrictions that are so severe that they require urgent hospital treatment. Regular massage to the neck and shoulder area can help reduce both the number and severity of asthma attacks. Massage can also be used to alleviate the symptoms of a mild attack.

a typical asthma profile

Asthma sufferers tend to be highly sensitive and particularly prone to stress and anxiety. Their breathing is rapid, shallow and restricted, with a tendency to breathe through the mouth rather than the nose.

pressure points on the back

The lung-associated acupressure point, situated on either side of the spine between the scapulae, is associated with relieving the symptoms of asthma and reducing muscle spasms in the shoulders and neck. Massage inbetween and around the shoulder blades can therefore help relax the muscles and give some relief during an asthma attack.

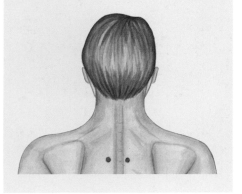

useful essential oils

These are some of the essential oils that help to open up the breathing, relax bronchial spasms and calm anxiety during a mild asthma attack. Use 2–3 drops essential oil added to 15ml (1 tbsp) massage oil or lotion, and use as a chest rub. Alternatively, vaporize the oils in a burner.
• eucalyptus or juniper: opens up the airways, encourages expulsion of mucus
• frankincense or marjoram: helps to calm and relax
• rosemary or peppermint: reduces general breathing difficulties

They are especially liable to hold tension in the neck, upper back and shoulders. Constriction in these areas inhibits the full expansion of the diaphragm, which in turn restricts lung capacity. Releasing tension in the neck and upper back through massage can help to open up the breathing. It can also help to calm anxiety and help the person to relax.

healthy breathing

Research has shown that there are some basic breathing principles that are especially helpful for asthmatics. The first is to develop the habit of breathing through the nose and not the mouth. Breathing through the nose helps to regulate and slow down the breathing. It also means that the air is warmed in the nasal passages before it enters the lungs. Cold air entering the lungs changes the chemical balance and can make the internal environment more susceptible to an asthma attack. Second, it is advised to try to breathe from the abdomen rather than the upper chest. This will help to slow down and deepen the breathing, which helps to stave off an oncoming attack.

causes and effects of asthma

Some types of asthma are triggered by an allergic response to dust, pollen and animal hair, as well as certain foodstuffs, such as dairy products. Other causative factors include stress and exposure to tobacco smoke and high levels of environmental pollution. There can also be cases where a genetic factor may also be involved.

During an asthma attack, the constricted bronchial passages cause wheezing, coughing, and feelings of panic, which serve to exacerbate the symptoms.

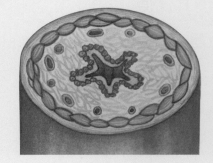

△ **Bronchial passages contract during an asthma attack as the surrounding muscles exert pressure on them, restricting breathing capacity.**

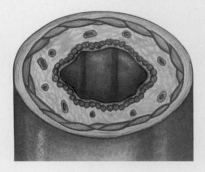

△ **When the attack has subsided and the muscles have relaxed, the airways can expand once more, allowing air to pass through unrestricted.**

massage for asthma

Have your partner sit at a table so they can lean forwards if they want or need to.

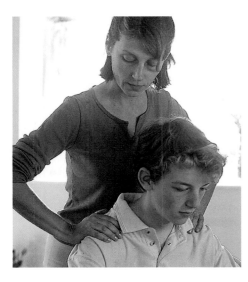

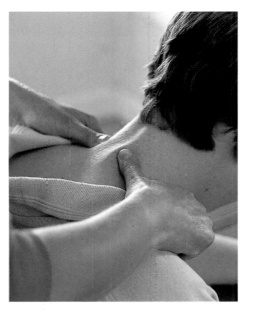

△ **3** Stand behind your partner and hold their shoulders, positioning your thumbs at the base of the neck. With both thumbs working together, make small firm circular strokes across the base of the neck (avoiding the spine), moving a little down into the upper back and a little up into the shoulders.

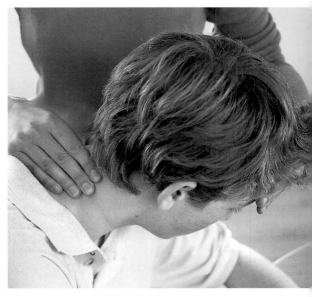

△ **4** Move to the left of your partner. Support their forehead with your left hand. Place your right hand at the base of the neck and, with a wide span, grasp and pull back the neck muscles. Sweep up to the middle and then to the top of the neck, using the same movement. Repeat three times.

△ **1** Gently place your hands on your partner's shoulders. Ask them to breathe in through their nose and then out for as long as possible. Do it with them. Ask them to take a second deep breath. On the out breath, gently press down on their shoulders encouraging them to soften.

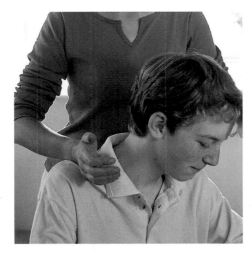

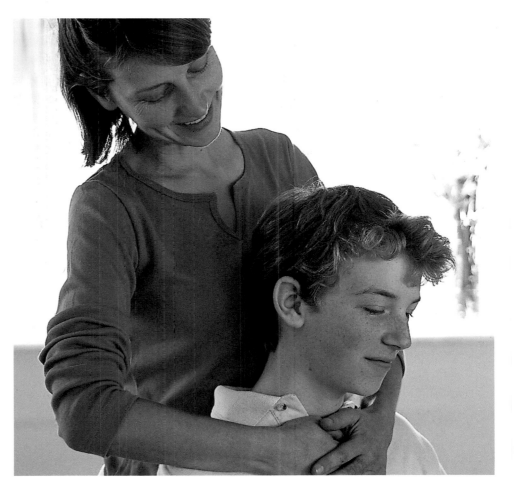

△ **2** Move a little to the left of your partner and anchor your left hand on their left shoulder. Holding your right hand loose and open, use a zigzag rubbing motion with the side of your hand, working along the top of your partner's right shoulder and then down around the shoulder blade into the back. Work the muscles that run inbetween the shoulder blade and the spine itself. Change sides and repeat.

△ **5** To finish the massage, put your hands on the front of your partner's chest just below the collarbone. Using a sweeping stroke, brush outwards and upwards towards the shoulders. Have a sense of your partner's chest opening and expanding as you work. Repeat three times. Come to a rest, putting your hands on your partner's shoulders and take a deep breath in and out together.

sense when the time is right to begin working on the massage sequence.

the other side. Use your fingers to firmly sweep out across the shoulders and down the back a few times.

from top to bottom. Repeat three times. Finish by gently stroking and pulling the earlobes.

Headache relief

There are many different types of headache, such as cluster headaches and migraines. However the vast majority of headaches are caused by muscular tension, with the pain ranging from mild to severe. Before rushing for the painkillers, try using a little head massage, as it is a very effective treatment for tension headaches. It not only eases the pain, but can also help re-educate the body so that it has a more relaxed response to stress and does not automatically tense up.

There are many reasons why muscular tension builds up, and tension headaches usually have a mixture of physical and psychological components. They often disappear once the stress trigger has gone. Where the trigger is ongoing however, the headaches can become chronic, with muscles locked in a state of contraction.

reflexology point for headaches

The pressure points that are most useful for headache treatments are those located at the base of the skull and the top of the spine. Make sure that when you are working on these points remain aware of how sensitive they are. Only apply very gentle pressure, and do not carry on if there is any pain or discomfort.

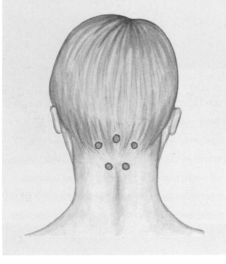

self-massage

The following strokes can be very effective for instant headache relief. They can be done almost anywhere. Leaning your elbows on the table and using your arms to provide support for your head makes the massage more effective.

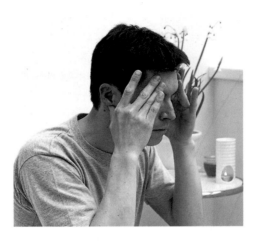

△ **1** Use the pads of your middle fingers to smooth out your forehead. Begin at the bottom of the brow area and work outwards, pressing and smoothing out towards the hairline. Then move your fingers up a little and work across the next section, continuing in this way until you have covered the whole forehead. Repeat twice more.

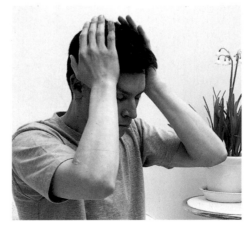

△ **2** Place your hands over your temples and press inwards with the heel of your hands (or use your palms if you prefer). Using a circling action, work six times in a clockwise direction and, reversing the movement, six times anti-clockwise.

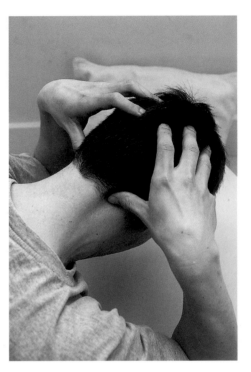

△ **3** Place your thumbs on the bony ridge behind your ears. Using a firm pressure, press and release. Continue with this action, working along the base of the skull until you get to the middle. Repeat three times. If you find any particularly tight spots, these are likely to be trigger points for the headache. Take a deep breath in, and on the out breath press more deeply, holding for a count of seven.

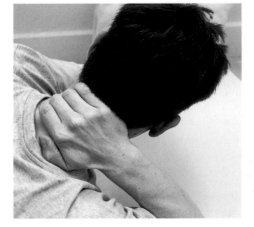

△ **4** Bend your head slightly forwards and support it with one hand. Use your other hand to clasp the back of your neck and squeeze it. Press as hard as you can and hold the pressure as you breathe out. Repeat so that the whole neck is worked over three times.

▷ To help your partner switch off and unwind, make sure the space you will be working in is relaxing and protecting. You should both feel comfortable and at ease.

massage with a partner

Head massage can help ease the pain of a tension headache. Where the headaches are chronic, regular treatments can also help dissolve deep-seated muscular tension and play a key role in ongoing stress management. Headache treatments are best done with your partner lying down so that their head is completely supported and the neck muscles have a chance to relax and let go. Make sure that your partner drinks plenty of water before and afterwards to encourage the elimination of toxins.

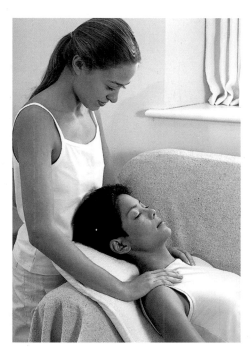

△ **1** Kneel at your partner's head and rest your hands over their shoulders. Ask your partner to take a deep breath in and out. On the out breath, gently press down on the shoulders, using both your hands. Repeat three times. This movement helps to relax tension in the shoulders, as well as releasing the muscles of the neck.

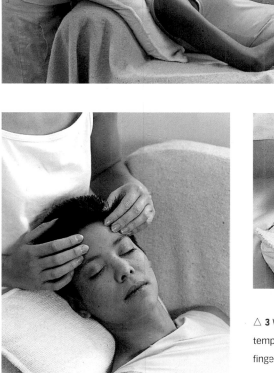

△ **2** Move your fingers to the middle of your partner's forehead. Keeping your fingers together, use smoothing strokes, working from the centre out towards the temples. Repeat several times. This relaxing movement helps to release tension in the tight muscles across the forehead.

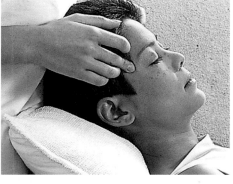

△ **3** With your hands positioned over your partner's temples, make small circular strokes with your fingertips. Check how much pressure feels good for your partner. If the headache is intense, a light touch is usually best. Move your fingers down and back slightly to continue the movement at the side of the skull just above the ears.

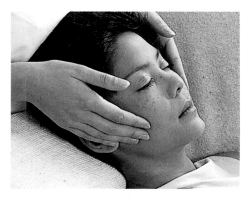

△ **4** Slide your hands down to the jaw hinge and continue to fingertip massage, using small circular strokes. Continue down the jaw line. The jaw holds a lot of tension and these strokes help it to release.

contraindications

Do not treat the following types of headaches with head massage: migraines and cluster headaches; those brought on by environmental factors such as noise or pollution, or by dehydration or exhaustion; and those associated with fever, illness, hangovers or infection.

Sinus decongestion

Sore sinuses can be extremely painful. They often follow in the wake of a cold or flu, but allergic conditions such as hay fever can also bring them on. The problem is caused by a build-up of mucus in the sinus cavities, which restricts the opening of the sinus into the nose. If the mucus membranes are inflamed or infected, the sinus area becomes very sore, and may give rise to headaches or facial pain. This condition is usually known as sinusitis. For mild cases or at the onset of an attack, massage can be extremely helpful in helping the mucus disperse and in relieving this distressing condition.

mucus production

The production of mucus is a primary response of the body's auto immune system. It is one of the body's first defences against pathogens (disease-causing agents), and is produced to destroy these hostile invaders. An increase in mucus could be in response to a virus, as in the case of coughs and colds. Or it could be an allergic reaction to substances such as tobacco smoke, pollen, chemicals, animal fur or certain foods. If an allergy is involved, it is advisable to try and identify the trigger and to eliminate it as far as possible.

acupressure points for sinus pain

Applying pressure to these acupressure points on the face and neck will help relieve sinus pain. If the area feels tender, only use the gentlest pressure.

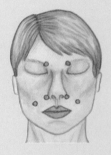

△ Use your ring fingers of both hands for these points on the face. Hold in position for a few seconds at a time.

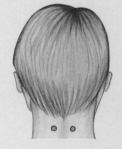

△ Acupressure points on the muscle either side of the spine just below the skull can help relieve congestion in the head. Apply gentle pressure on them with your thumbs.

steam inhalations

A steam inhalation can work wonders, particularly after a massage when the mucus has been loosened. You need a towel, a bowl of hot water and maybe one or two essential oils. Eucalyptus and peppermint have anti-viral, cleansing and head-clearing properties, while lavender is anti-viral and a relaxant. Add 2–3 drops of oil to the hot water. Use the towel to make a tent over your head and the bowl, close your eyes and breathe in the steam. If you suffer from asthma, steam inhalations are best avoided.

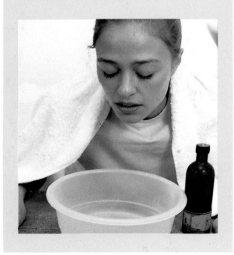

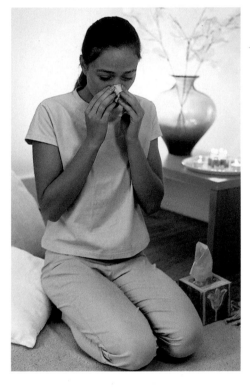

△ If you are suffering from congestion try to eliminate dairy products, sugar and wheat from your diet as these foods are all mucus forming. Increasing your fluid intake by drinking more water, herbal teas or hot ginger and lemon will also help the body to flush out congestion.

▷ When facial sinus points are too sensitive or painful to touch, the sides of the fingertips provide an alternative place to exert gentle pressure, using your thumb and index finger.

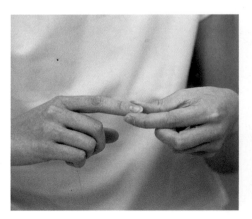

self-massage for sinus relief

Congested sinuses are often painful to touch, so working on yourself allows you to regulate the level of pressure. This routine can be done a number of times through the day to help clear congestion and assist breathing. Ideally, this massage should be followed by a steam inhalation with essential oils to help flush out the mobilized congestion.

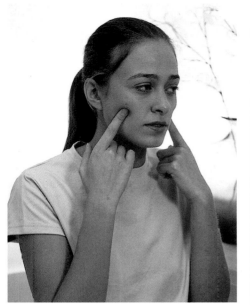

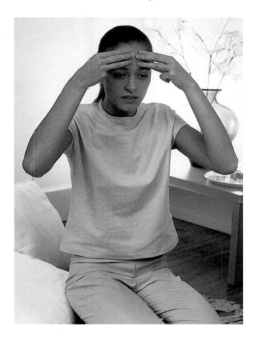

△ **1** Sit in a comfortable position and place your hands just above the mid-point between the eyebrows. Work your way across the forehead, making small circles with your fingertips. Anchor your thumbs at the temples and stretch your fingers to meet in the middle of the forehead. Then sweep your fingers out and across the forehead, imagining your sinuses clearing out as you do so. Use whatever pressure is comfortable.

contraindication

Massage is contraindicated in sinus conditions that are accompanied by a fever, green or yellow mucus, or that have been going on for more than three days. In these cases you should seek medical advice.

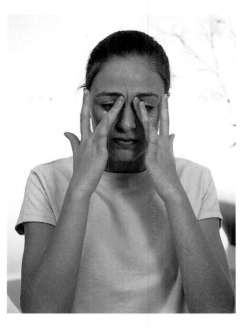

△ **2** Place your middle fingers in the spot on either side of the nose where it meets the underside of the eyebrows. Take a breath in, and on the out breath, press firmly for a few seconds and then release. Repeat three times. This is a crucial pressure point for the sinuses and may feel tender to touch. Continue along the underside of both eyebrows for about 2.5cm (1in), exerting similar pressure. The sequence is press, hold, release, repeat and move on. Complete by using a pinch-and-lift movement on the eyebrows, working your way along to the outside edge. Repeat a few times.

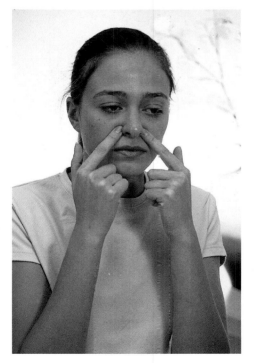

△ **3** Position your index fingers on either side at the base of the nose and apply pressure, holding and then releasing. Repeat three times. This is another important pressure point for opening up the sinuses.

△ **4** Draw your fingers out along the underside of the cheekbones and use pressure strokes along its edge. A sinus drainage tube runs along this area. There are more drainage points underneath the jawbone, running from the middle of the chin to the ear. Use your thumbs to make small circular movements along this line. Finish with some smooth sliding strokes that will help to drain away the congestion.

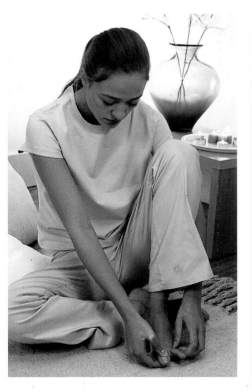

△**5** For maximum effect, or if the sinus areas are too painful, you can work with foot pressure points. Squeeze and press the tips of your toes and press and slide down their sides to the pads beneath. Continue doing this, paying particular attention to the big toes. To relieve a frontal sinus headache, apply pressure to just below the nail of the big toe.

Sensual massage

Touch is the language of lovers and enjoying massage with your partner adds another dimension to your relationship, becoming part of your intimate exchange and a special way of spending time together. Head massage can be given in such a way that it becomes a sensual experience. Although some of the strokes in a sensual head massage are different from those in the standard routine, the key feature is the sensual quality of your touch and the blending of your energies together. It can be done with or without oils.

mood setting

To set the scene for a romantic and intimate space, think soft and warm. Candles, cushions and an open fire are traditional favourites for creating the right atmosphere; if you don't have an open fire turn up the heating. Use your creative flair to beautify the space with flowers, fabrics and background music. You could also light some incense or vaporize essential oils in a burner. Many fragrances have sensual, aphrodisiac qualities – some of the most popular include sandalwood, jasmine, ylang ylang, rose and patchouli. Have plenty of towels and warm coverings to hand and a comfortable surface to work on. A duvet, futon, blankets or soft sheepskins make a well-padded surface. Finally, wear something loose and comfortable and appropriate to the romantic occasion.

giving sensual massage

If you are tense it will be difficult for your partner to relax, so make sure you keep your jaw and shoulders soft and breathe from your belly. Focus on giving pleasure to your partner by tuning in to their breathing and being sensitive to their changing responses. Enjoy making your strokes long and lingering or firmer and more stimulating, using your judgement and spontaneity as you work. The massage can be done sitting up or lying down.

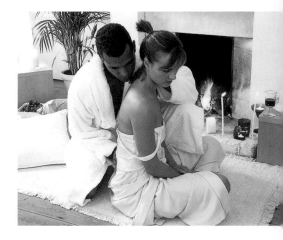

△ **1** This stroke stimulates the release and flow of sexual energy from the sacrum at the base of the spine. Place one hand on your partner's shoulder and the other at the base of the spine. Using your fingertips and very light pressure, make circular strokes in a clockwise direction around the sacrum. Build up a smooth rhythm and make the circles larger till the whole back is circled, each time returning to the sacrum. Gradually decrease their size, finishing at the sacrum.

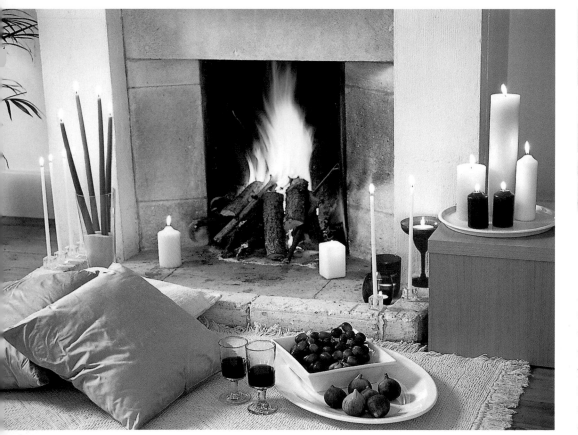

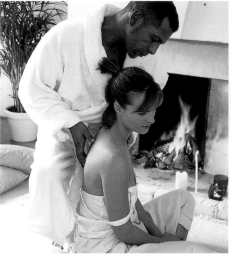

△ **2** With one hand on your partner's head, gently draw the fingers of your working hand up their back to the base of the neck. From here, gently stroke up the back of the neck a couple of times. If you wish you may also blow soft circles of warm air on the back of the neck. Both of these actions stimulate the nerve receptors in the skin and should send shivers of pleasure up your partner's spine.

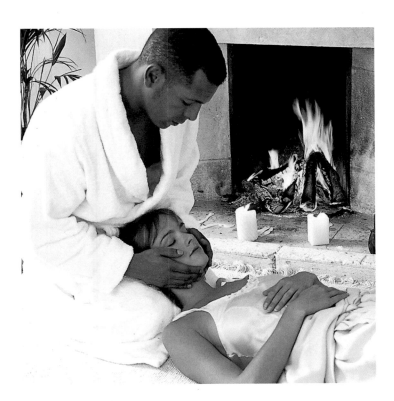

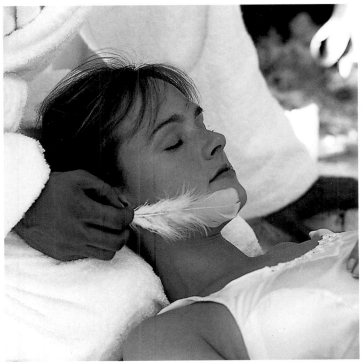

△ **3** For work on the face, your partner may prefer to lie down. Find a comfortable position with their head cradled on your lap or on a cushion. Place your hands at the bottom of their face so that you are cupping their chin. Slowly and gently draw your hands up over the face, up to the forehead and then stroke back down the sides to the chin. Repeat five times. To extend this stroke, use one finger to trace the features of your partner's face, beginning at the lips, and moving up around the nose, cheeks, eye sockets and eyebrows. Trace each feature three times.

△ **5** Use a feather (or your own hair if it is long enough) for this stroke. Beginning at the chin, slowly trail the feather up the side of the face with slow luxurious strokes. Return to the chin and repeat several times and then switch sides. You can also stroke across the cheekbones and brow, working from the middle out towards the hairline each time. Imagine you are caressing away all cares and tensions as you lovingly stroke. Repeat several times. Should your partner find this ticklish, substitute the feather with some lingering finger stroking up and across the face.

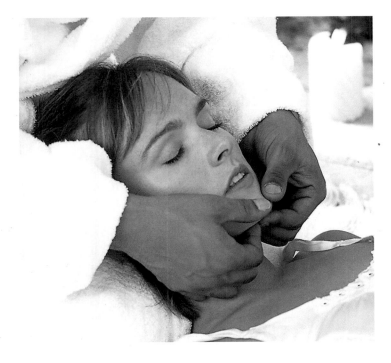

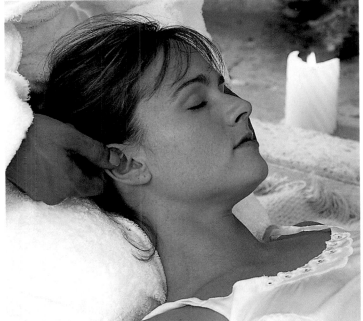

△ **4** Place both thumbs in the middle of your partner's chin, with the index fingers curled underneath. Make small circles with your thumbs on the chin, underneath the mouth and a little out into the lower cheeks, using your fingers underneath for support. As you work, make the circles slightly bigger to include the lower lip. Then gently use your thumbs to pull the lower lip down so that the lips are slightly open. To extend this stroke, continue to make small circular strokes with the pads of your fingers all over the face and forehead. Use a light touch and avoid the eye area.

△ **6** Holding your partner's earlobes between your thumb and fingers, gently massage the ears by squeezing and rolling, moving up along each ear's outside edge and then down on the inside edge. Continue working round the ears until you have completed three laps. Then, using your ring finger, trace round each ear's outside and top edge as well as its' inside surface. This is a highly delicate area, but done sensitively it can feel very intimate and sensual. Finish by gently pulling down on the earlobes a couple of times.

Babies and children

It is never too soon to enjoy massage. In many parts of the world, it is customary for babies and children to be massaged by their mothers and carers. Touch is a natural expression of love, communicating warmth and security. In babies, massage helps strengthen the growing bond between mother and baby. Babies also enjoy it and usually sleep better afterwards. Children too are generally receptive to being massaged. The important thing to remember when working with babies or children is that their bodies are still developing so they must be treated very gently.

massage for babies

When giving baby massage, focus on the chest and back, using light, smooth strokes. Do NOT massage the head, as this is too malleable. The best time to massage your baby is at the end of the day, before feeding and bathing. Although it may be the last thing you feel like doing, once you start you'll find it relaxes you both. If at any point you sense your baby is not enjoying the massage, then stop. The massage should only go on if you are both enjoying it.

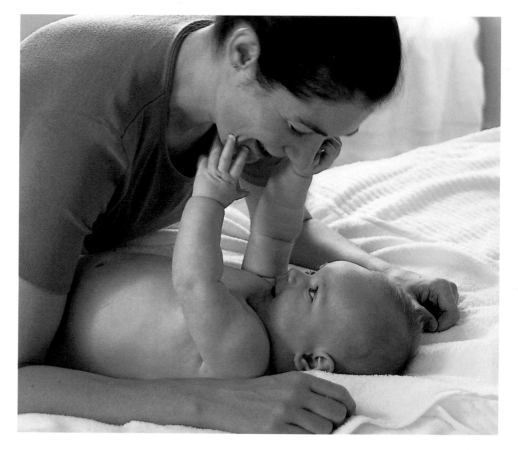

△ Begin a massage by looking into the baby's eyes and establishing a connection. Keep in contact and let intuition be your guide.

preparation and massage

Make sure the room is warm, as babies feel the cold, and their body temperatures can drop quickly. Have a soft cloth or towel for your baby to lie on and, if you are using oil, warm it up before applying. In India, a blend of coconut and sesame oil is often used in baby massage, although almond, apricot or grape seed oils are also suitable. Ideally the oil should be cold-pressed and organic.

Begin by playing with your baby, talking and looking into their eyes to establish contact. Then pour a little oil into your hands and rub it in gently, using circular movements on the baby's chest.

After a minute or so, sit your baby up and massage the back, stroking in a criss-cross motion, making sure you cover the whole area. Then, using your fingertips, make little circular strokes up and down the back, avoiding the spine. Move to the shoulders, and stroke over this area and then down the length of the back before drawing to a close.

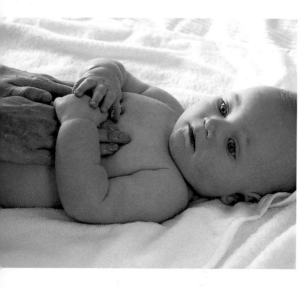

△ Begin the massage of your baby by stroking with the whole of your hand on the chest. Use both hands and make smooth, gentle, circular movements. Keep eye contact all the time.

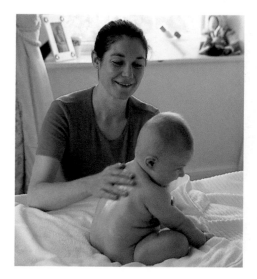

△ To massage your baby's back, either lie him down across your knees or sit him up with your hand supporting his chest. Stroke up and down the back in a criss-cross motion.

▷ You can do head massage or children from when they are aged about three years old. It is best to keep treatments light, short and sweet at this tender age.

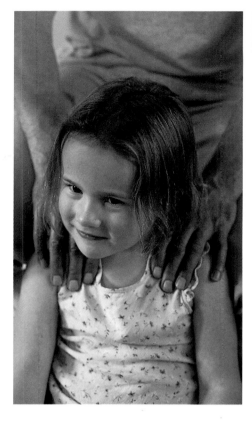

children and modern society

Today's children probably have more complications and stresses in their lives than their counterparts of a generation or two ago. From a young age, they can be expected to cope with many difficult situations, such as divorce, academic pressures and complex lifestyle patterns. They spend more time in sedentary activities, such as watching television or using the computer, with less time in physical pursuits, which would help to release stress naturally, as well as keeping the child fit and strong. Many children are becoming obese and are developing poor postural habits, which will cause them problems in later life. It can also be difficult for older children to show their feelings. Head massage can help with many of these difficulties. It can release physical tension, provide both emotional and psychological support, as well as helping to correct some important postural imbalances.

▽ It is never too early for your baby to begin enjoying the benefits of massage. Starting gentle massage at an early age will pay dividends later on.

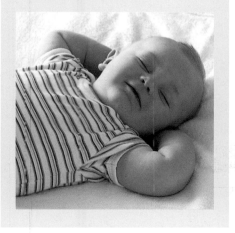

massage for children

When your massage partner is a younger child, you will probably need to find a higher chair, such as a kitchen stool, for them to sit on. You can also use cushions to raise the seat. Make sure the child's legs are not left dangling by using cushions under their feet. Be flexible and creative in your approach, giving appropriate treatment when called for: you can offer a back or shoulder rub for instance if the child complains of a headache. A treatment that lasts between 5–10 minutes is usually sufficient. Be sensitive to how the child reacts, and don't try to persuade them to continue if they get restless or ill at ease.

When massaging teenagers, remember that they don't always welcome physical contact, and keep the massage as relaxed and informal as you can. Don't over-prepare the situation; take the opportunity when it comes to suggest a massage as part of your usual interaction with each other.

▽ It is all too easy to overlook the fact that young people experience stress in their bodies much the same as adults do, and that regular massage helps them enormously.

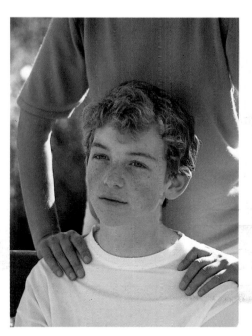

At the end of a massage with a young person, stand behind them and put both your hands on their shoulders, fingers pointing forwards. Ask them to take a deep breath in and out. On the second out breath, gently press down with your hands and then let go. This helps to "ground" their energy and to release any remaining tension.

▽ Children learn by experience, and by receiving massage they can soon learn how to become proficient masseurs themselves, as happens in other parts of the world.

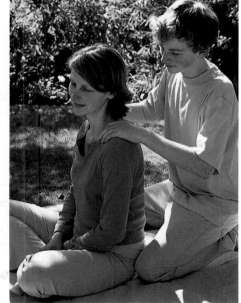

Head massage for insomnia and illness

Massage can give comfort to someone who is unwell and accelerate the healing process, and for sleep-related problems it can relax the body and help the mind to switch off. These very different situations require different approaches.

treating insomnia

For chronic sleeplessness the underlying causes need to be investigated, but generally most sleep problems are linked to stress and tension. When you're lying in bed and can't get to sleep, you can use head massage to ease body tension and hopefully induce calm and peaceful slumber. The strokes are suitable for both partner and self-massage.

To prepare yourself breathe deeply in and out from your belly, perhaps letting out a sigh or a yawn on the out breath. Then let your jaw drop so that your mouth is partly open and your tongue rests softly in it. Roll up a small ball of saliva in your mouth and keep it there – higher levels of body fluid are associated with deeper states of relaxation. Keep your eyes gently closed, making sure that your eye sockets remain soft. Keep your mouth moist with saliva.

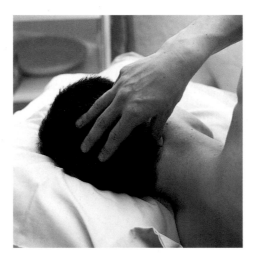

△ **2** Still lying on your side, use your thumb to press into the base of the skull in the area just behind the ear. Continue pressing, moving down along the skull's ridge to the hollow in the middle of its base. Stay longer in any particularly tight or painful spots. You can also make circular strokes here with your thumbs. There are many pressure points along this area that can help to promote restful sleep. Turn your head and repeat on the other side.

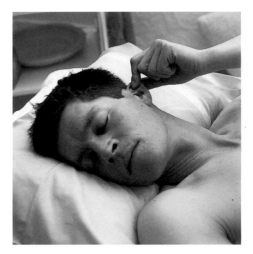

△ **4** Turning your head slightly, place your ring finger at the top of your upper ear. Slide it down to just below the ear's top outer ridge and across to the edge of the dimple in this ridge. Position your thumb so that it is resting on the underside of the ear's ridge, just behind your ring finger. Press firmly and use your finger to massage in a circular movement for about 30 seconds. This special pressure point is associated with calming the mind. Repeat on the other ear.

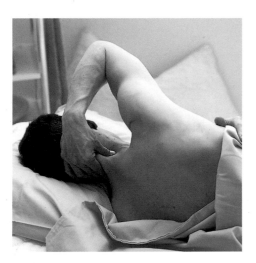

△ **1** As you breathe out, firmly squeeze the middle back of your neck with one hand. Hold the pressure for 15 seconds and slowly release. Repeat at the top and bottom of your neck. Cover the neck area three times and repeat on other side.

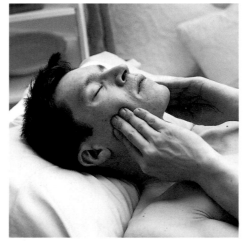

△ **3** Now lie on your back, and use your fingers to make circling strokes around the jaw area, paying particular attention to the jaw socket. Use stronger pressure here if you wish. As the jaw benefits from repetitive work, keep this action going for a few minutes. As you massage you can listen to the soothing sound of your breath. Alternatively, breathe in through your nose and out through your mouth to encourage repetitive, sleep-inducing yawning.

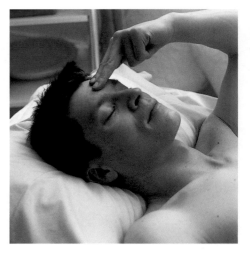

△ **5** With your head back to centre, place your two middle fingers in the middle of your forehead and make slow circular strokes using a light pressure. Continue with this circling action and work out towards your right temple, making the circles bigger as you go. Circle over the temple area and then use connecting circular strokes to move to the left temple. Repeat once or twice more. This stroke also calms the mind and slows down thinking processes.

▷ **A soothing presence of touch can be very reassuring and pleasurable to receive when feeling unwell and can help accelerate healing.**

head massage and illness

During illness, a traditional style head massage would be over-stimulating and could feel invasive. The body's energies are taken up with trying to get well and in these situations a different kind of approach is called for. A gentle hand massage that uses light and tender strokes, however, can be healing and soothing to receive and also speed up recovery. This type of massage can be used during convalescence but not during acute conditions. Before massaging anyone who is unwell, observe the usual contraindications; if you have any doubt then check with a qualified medical practitioner. As a general guide, remember to keep your touch light and gentle and avoid firm pressure. The strokes should be fluid, smooth and flowing and stop when your partner has had enough.

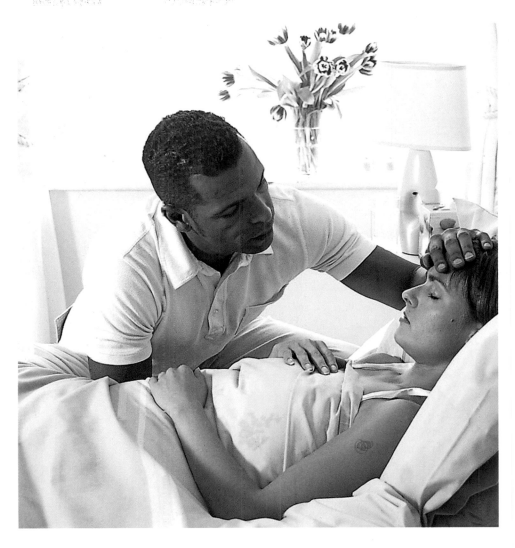

hand massage

A light hand massage can promote healing and relaxation throughout the body's systems without being too vigorous. Pressure points on the hand have physiological correspondences to the rest of the body, there are also nerve receptors located here which will send messages of relaxation to the brain.

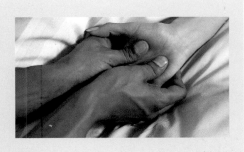

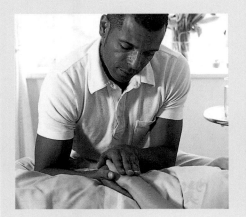

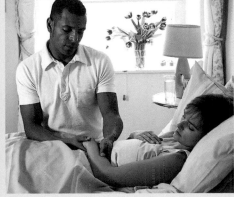

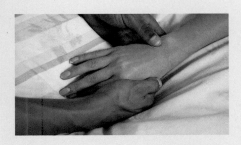

3△ Using your thumb pads, make small circular strokes across the whole palm at least three times, including the wrist area if you wish.

1△ Gently sandwich your partner's hand in between your hands and then use your top hand to stroke downwards in the direction of the fingertips. Next, take each finger at a time and stroke down to the fingertip. Repeat on each finger three times. Repeat on the other hand.

2△ Next, move your hands to the arm and make circling actions with your thumbs, working round the muscles of the arm, then the joints of the wrist and hand. Make your touch increasingly light as you move down the arm. Do this three times and then change to the other arm.

4△ Make light circular strokes over the front of the hand, working gently into the wrist and smoothing between the fingers. Finish with gentle stroking and a hold. Repeat on the other hand.

Oil Massage for Health and Beauty

Plant oils have been used for healing and cosmetic purposes for thousands of years. Certain oils not only nourish and improve the condition of the hair, skin and scalp, but because they are absorbed through the skin into the bloodstream, they can have a positive effect on health and wellbeing throughout the body's systems.

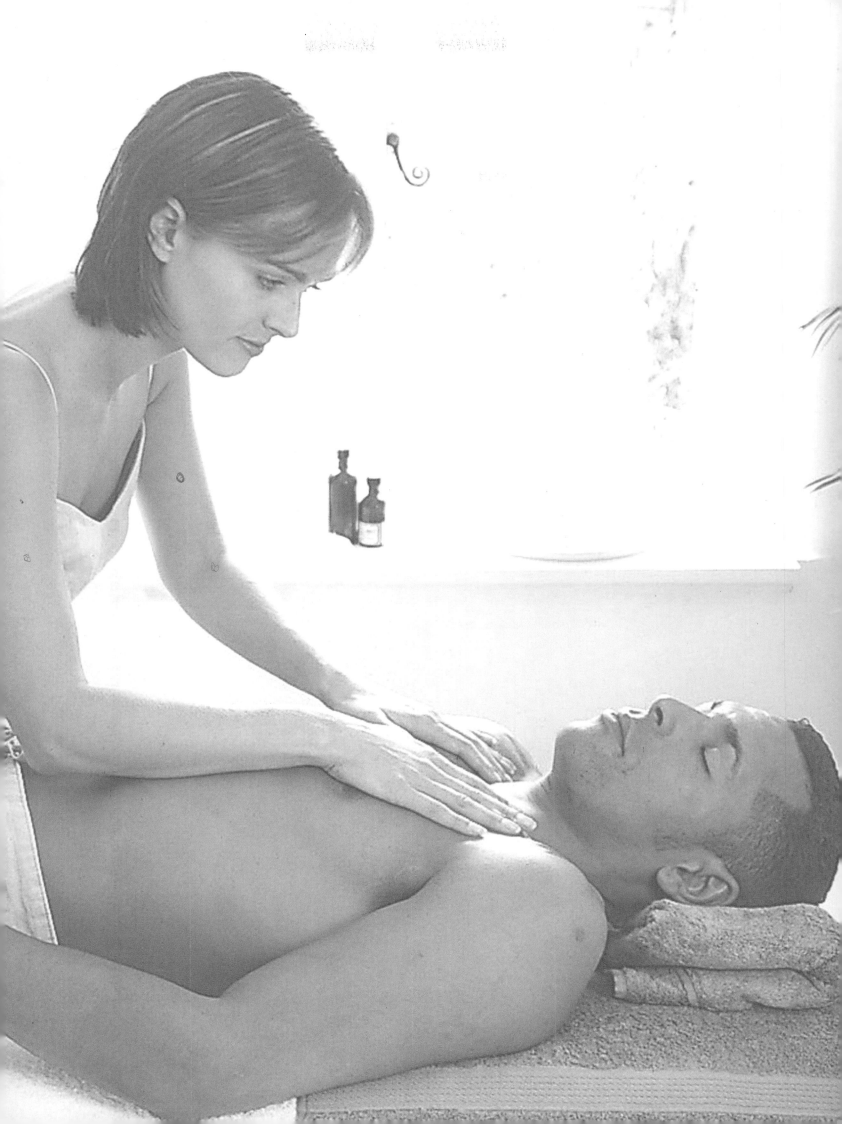

Using oils in head massage

There are many benefits of using oil in head massage, the most obvious being the conditioning effect on the hair and scalp itself. The effects of stress, chemical hair treatments, central heating and poor nutrition can all be seen in the health of our hair and scalp. Similarly, frequent hair washing and the use of hairdryers and heated hair-styling devices strip the hair of its natural oils, making it dry and brittle. Using oils can help restore the hair to its optimum condition, penetrating deep into the hair shaft to strengthen the hair. Unlike most ready-made products they do not contain any harsh detergents or chemicals and can be custom-blended to suit your specific needs. There is a wide array of suitable oils for use in head massage. These fall into two broad categories: carrier oils and essential oils.

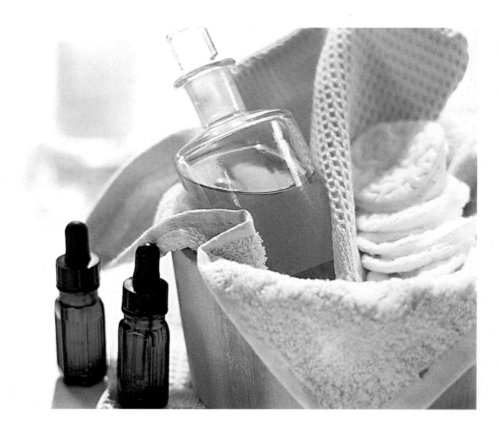

carrier oils

Traditionally, carrier oils are used in their own right in head massage, but they can also be used as a base to mix with essential oils. Sweet almond is one of the most versatile carrier oils. It is easily absorbed and is a warming, light oil. It can help reduce muscular pain and stiffness.

In Ayurveda, sesame oil is very popular for massaging the head and body. It helps to strengthen, condition and moisturize the skin and hair. It is a balancing oil and can help to reduce swelling, pain and stiffness.

Deep yellow mustard oil is thick and heavy. Its strong characteristic odour makes it unsuitable for blending with essential oils, so only use it by itself. Mustard oil has a stimulating effect on the circulatory system, helping to increase body heat and warm up the muscles and joints. Its properties help to ease general aches and pains, tension and

△ **Using oils as part of your regular beauty routine can be of lasting benefit in helping you to keep looking and feeling good.**

swellings. It is a good oil to use in the cold winter months or when the body is chilled. Another thick and warming oil that can ease muscular pain and stiffness is olive oil. Use the best quality virgin, extra virgin or cold-pressed oils as these contain high levels of unsaturated fatty acids that are nourishing for dry skin and hair.

Light coconut oil is used extensively in southern India. It is easy to use and blends well with essential oils. It has softening and moisturizing qualities that makes it ideal for dry, brittle or chemically-treated hair. You can also leave it on the hair to give a high gloss sheen or "wet look".

Finally, luxurious jojoba oil is rich in protein, minerals and vitamin E. It is ideal for use on all skin and hair types and mixes well with essential oils. Because it is expensive, jojoba is usually used in a mix with another carrier oil.

▽ **Used regularly in traditional Indian head massage, light coconut oil, sweet almond oil and sesame oil have therapeutic properties.**

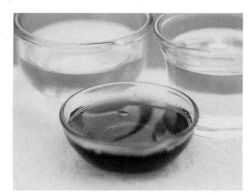

▽ **Olive oil has been used in skin treatments for centuries in the Mediterranean region for its nourishing properties and versatility.**

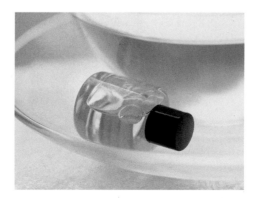

▷ A relaxing bath fragranced with essential oils will round off a head massage. Alternatively, it will help you to fully unwind at the end of a long and tiring day.

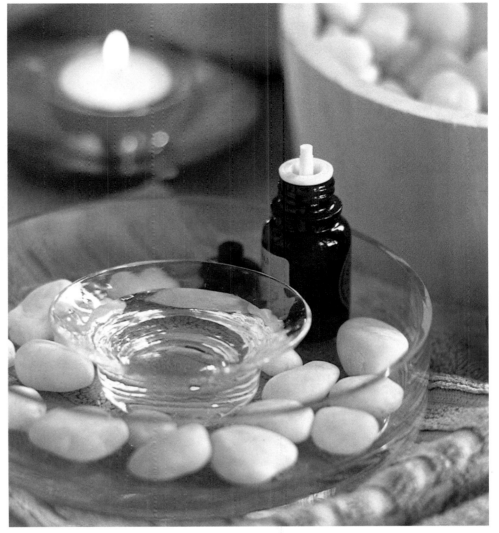

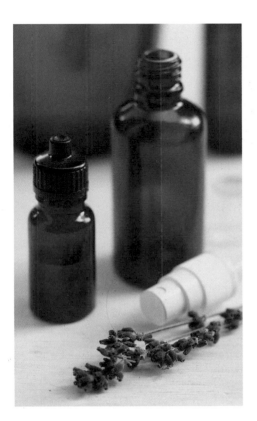

△ Lavender oil is the most popular essential oil in the West because of its wide variety of uses for both young and old alike.

essential oils

Highly concentrated plant oils are known as "essential" oils. These potent oils have a complex chemistry and a strong distinctive aroma, and affect the body on a physical, mental and emotional level. Essential oils are never used directly, but are blended with a carrier oil to achieve a specific therapeutic effect. The following oils are particularly suitable for head massage.

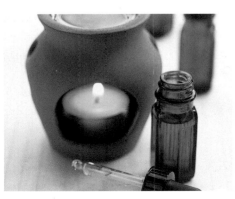

lavender One of the most universal of all the essential oils, lavender's relaxing and balancing properties make it useful for stress, insomnia, anxiety and depression. It is useful for treating dandruff, hair loss and lice and blends well with geranium and rosemary.

rosemary The refreshing and stimulating properties of rosemary oil have a head-clearing effect, so it is useful for periods of mental work. Rosemary is also a good treatment for greasy hair and skin, dandruff and hair loss, as well as restoring the shine to dark hair. It blends well with lavender.

sandalwood This oil's woody, haunting aroma quietens the mind and relaxes the nervous system, making it useful for stress-related conditions. Its softening and soothing action is good for dry skin and scalp conditions, while its aphrodisiac properties

◁ Using essential oils in a burner will enhance the ambience of the space you work in and help transport you to another dimension.

lend itself to sensual massage. Sandalwood blends well with bergamot, cedarwood, jasmine, palmarosa, vetiver or ylang ylang.

frankincense This has calming and relaxing properties for body, mind and soul. Because it deepens and slows down breathing, frankincense is good for respiratory conditions such as asthma, blocked sinuses, coughs or colds. Its moisturizing properties make it especially nourishing for older skin. Frankincense has a tradition of use in sacred ceremony and is helpful for inner journeys or process of change.

geranium A light floral fragrance with a refreshing and balancing action, it is used to normalize very dry or very greasy skin and hair conditions by bringing them back into balance. Emotionally it is calming, restoring, uplifting and useful for anxiety or depression. It is an oil to use if you are uncertain which to choose. It blends well with lavender, sandalwood, rose, bergamot, marjoram, lemon or orange.

Working with oils

Oils are messy to work with so you need to make sure your partner is not wearing anything that could be spoiled – an old t-shirt is ideal. Keep a couple of towels specifically for this purpose and drape one around your partner's shoulders. Have a good supply of tissues to hand and gather together all your oils, plus a suitable spoon and mixing bowl. Put the equipment on absorbent paper to soak up any accidental spills. You will also need a shower cap or silver foil to wrap your partner's hair up in when you've finished. If your partner has long hair, it is best to apply oil in sections over the head, in which case you will also need a comb, tinting brush and hair clips.

using essential oils

Essential oils are highly potent and should be used sparingly. They are not used directly on the skin but are blended with a suitable carrier. Use in a ratio of 2 drops essential oil to every 10ml (2 tsp) carrier oil.

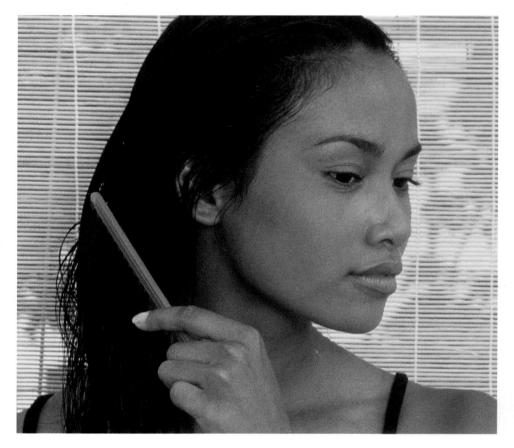

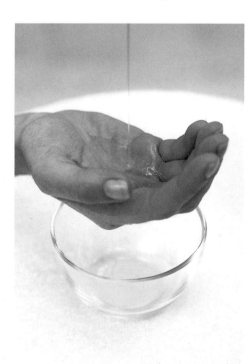

△ Warm the oil up in the palm of your hand or on a radiator before applying it, as heated oil is more easily absorbed and feels nicer.

△ Leaving the oils in your hair after an oil massage is a holistic treatment and helps leave your hair and scalp in excellent condition.

Exceeding the recommended dose could result in toxicity. Sometimes essential oils can cause allergic skin reactions. If you are using an oil for the first time, it is a good idea to do a patch test by dabbing a little of the blended oil on the inside of the wrist or elbow. Wait for 24 hours to see if there is any adverse reaction before using the oil.

Because of their potent effect, do not use essential oils with babies, young children or in pregnancy. When treating older children or the elderly, it is best to halve the dilution to 1 drop essential oil to every 10ml (2 tsp) carrier. If you are in doubt, consult a qualified aromatherapist.

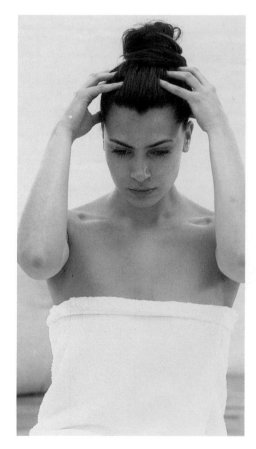

▷ Applying nourishing oils to your hair as part of your weekly beauty routine can be combined with a relaxing head massage.

oils for the hair and scalp

Choose from the following recipes to give your hair and scalp a nourishing conditioning treatment.

normal hair

carrier oils: almond, coconut, jojoba
essential oils: rosemary, lavender, geranium

dandruff

carrier oils: jojoba, olive, coconut, sweet almond
essential oils: rosemary, lavender, eucalyptus, geranium

greasy hair

carrier oils: sweet almond, sesame, jojoba
essential oils: rosemary, lavender, sandalwood, lemon

thinning hair

carrier oils: sesame, olive
essential oils: rosemary, lavender, geranium

dry or chemically-treated hair

carrier oils: sesame, coconut, jojoba, almond
essential oils: lavender, rosemary, geranium, sandalwood

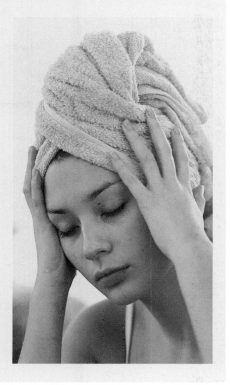

hair and scalp treatments

Mixing up your own blends of oils for your treatments is both very satisfying and beneficial. It is empowering and you can also ensure that the ingredients you are putting on your hair and scalp are fresh and potent (all the oils have a limited shelf life) and are of a high quality. Because you are choosing the raw ingredients you can guarantee that the blend you make is appropriate and of nutritional benefit to your body. Choose a carrier oil and an essential oil or two from the category on the left that best describes your hair. As a rough guide, 10ml (2 tsp) carrier oil should be sufficient for short hair, 15ml (1 tbsp) for medium length hair, and 30ml (2 tbsp) for long hair. The amount of oil you will need will also depend on the texture and thickness of the hair.

Measure the carrier oil into the mixing bowl. You may use more than one carrier oil if you wish, but mix them well together. Next add your chosen essential oil/s. Try not to make up more than you think you'll need, as it is best to work with a fresh mix each time. If you do have any left over, you could rub it into areas of rough skin, such as the elbows or heels. To get the most from the treatment, leave the oils on the hair for as long as possible, from a minimum of 30 minutes to up to 12 hours.

treating head lice

Head lice (nits) are a common problem among school-age children, and they can be difficult to eradicate. Using essential oils is becoming a popular treatment, as it offers a natural rather than a chemical approach to the problem. When treating lice it is essential that the whole family is treated to prevent the risk of cross-infection, and that all bedding, clothes, combs and brushes are washed to remove the eggs.

The quantity given below is sufficient for one complete treatment for one person. It comprises three separate applications, so you will have to store the remainder of the mixture in a sealed dark glass jar or bottle. It will keep for up to 12 months.

Use 30ml (2 tbsp) coconut or almond oil (or a combination of the two if you prefer). Add 9 drops lavender, 9 drops geranium and 9 drops eucalyptus oil. Apply the mix all over the head and hair, massaging it in well. Cover the head and leave the oils in for a minimum of 4 hours, although overnight is better. To remove the oil, massage the shampoo well into the hair before applying water. Wash and rinse as normal. Comb through the hair with a lice comb. Repeat the whole process after 24 hours and again after 8 days. This will give you the opportunity to treat any lice that have hatched since the first treatment and to ensure the head is clear.

▽ **Oil treatments can be therapeutic, and the treatment of head lice with oil blends is very effective, toxic-free and pleasant.**

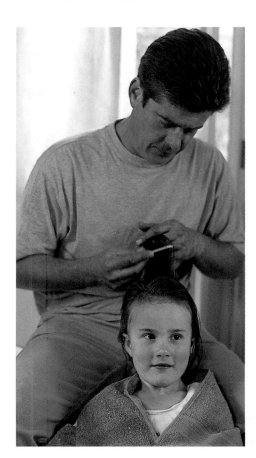

How to apply oils

The tradition of anointing the head with oil dates back to antiquity. There are many references to the practice throughout the Bible, while it has always played an important part in Ayurvedic medicine. In India, the practice of putting oil on the head begins at birth when a piece of soft cloth soaked in oil is placed over the fontanelle (the "soft spot") on a newborn baby's head. There are also complex ritual procedures within Ayurveda for applying oils to the head. Today traditional methods for applying oils have been integrated into a style more suited to a Western approach. Oil can be applied with your partner lying on a couch or sitting upright on a chair. Whichever method you use, warm the oil first. Warm oil not only feels nicer but it is more easily absorbed by the hair and scalp. To warm the oil, place it in a bowl on top of a radiator, or in a pan of hot water. Make sure the oil is not too hot before putting it on your partner's head. Take some time to discuss with your partner which oils and aromas they prefer, let them sniff the bottles and together work out a mix that will suit their state of mind and preferences.

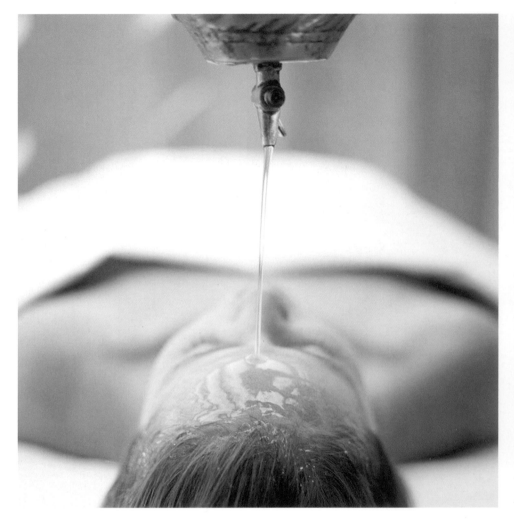

△ In Ayurvedic medicine the calming treatment of slowly and steadily pouring warmed oil over the forehead soothes and uplifts the spirit.

◁ Choosing which oils to use is part of the session and it is a good idea to discuss any preferences with your partner before starting.

lying-down method

Cover the surface of a couch or bed with suitable towels and have your partner lie down with their head near the edge. It's also a good idea to put a towel on the floor immediately below your partner's head.

Pour a little of the warmed oil directly on to the crown of your partner's head – it is a wonderful feeling as the oil seeps across the scalp. If you prefer, you may find it easier to pour some oil into the palm of your hand

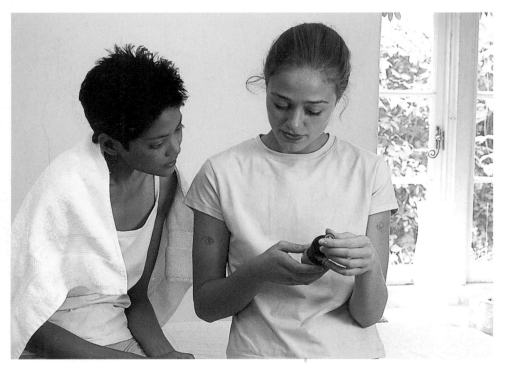

▷ Make sure you have assembled everything and that it is to hand before you begin working with oils, as they can be messy.

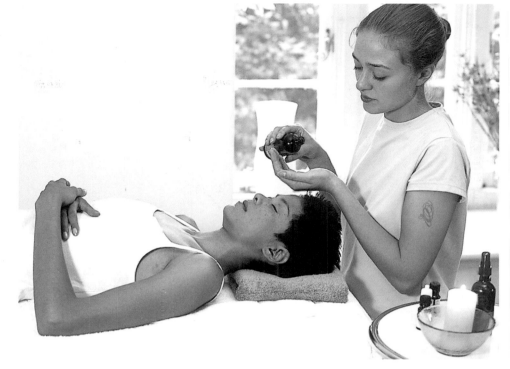

and put it on top of your partner's head like that. Work the oil into the scalp, applying more oil should you need to.

Pour more oil into your palm and massage up from the sides of the head towards the top. Put some more oil in your hand and apply it to the front of their head and work it upwards towards the middle. Then apply oil to the back of the head. Make sure that you have covered the whole head with oil. You can use this method with your partner sitting in a chair too. You are then ready to proceed with the same head massage routine described earlier. The strokes are the same; the only difference is the presence of the oil.

▽ Use your hands to apply a little oil into the hair at a time, working it well into the hair and scalp for a nourishing treatment.

sectioning method

This method divides the head into sections and is particularly suitable for longer hair. In addition to the oil you will need some hair clips and a comb.

Using the hair clips, divide the head into roughly eight sections, pinning the hair up and out of the way. Then, starting at the front of the head, take down one section of hair and comb the oil through, beginning at the roots and working all the way down to the hair ends. Take down another section and repeat. Continue until the whole head is covered, then proceed with your head massage sequence.

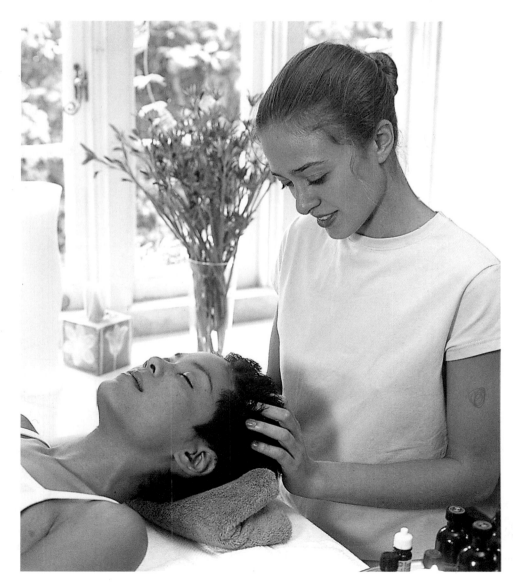

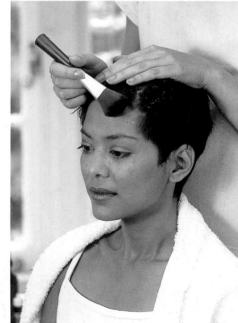

leaving and removing oils

To get the most out of an oil treatment the oils are best left on the head for some time. This maximizes their beneficial effects, giving them a chance to sink into the hair shaft and nourish it at a deep level. They will also be absorbed through the skin and enter the bloodstream where they will work their benefits through the whole body. Oils can be left on the hair from anything from 20 minutes to 24 hours. When it is time to remove them, there are a few guidelines for leaving your hair grease-free.

leaving oils on the hair

Once you have put the oils on, you will need to cover up your head. This will trap body heat and help the oils sink further into the hair and scalp. It may also feel more comfortable, particularly if you have long hair. You can do this by wearing a shower cap or by covering the head with silver foil, and bending it round at the corners to form a cap. You can then wrap a towel round your head to keep warm.

If you are keeping the oils on for an evening, then the treatment can be made part of a general pampering session combining self- or partner massage and other "feel-good" treats, such as a relaxing aromatherapy bath. Alternatively, leaving the oils in overnight will provide your hair and scalp with a deep conditioning treatment.

▽ **Leaving oils on your hair gives them a chance to sink in and deeply condition while you relax and take some quality time out.**

△ **For a really deep conditioning treatment, oils can be left on overnight and can continue working while you recharge with a restful sleep.**

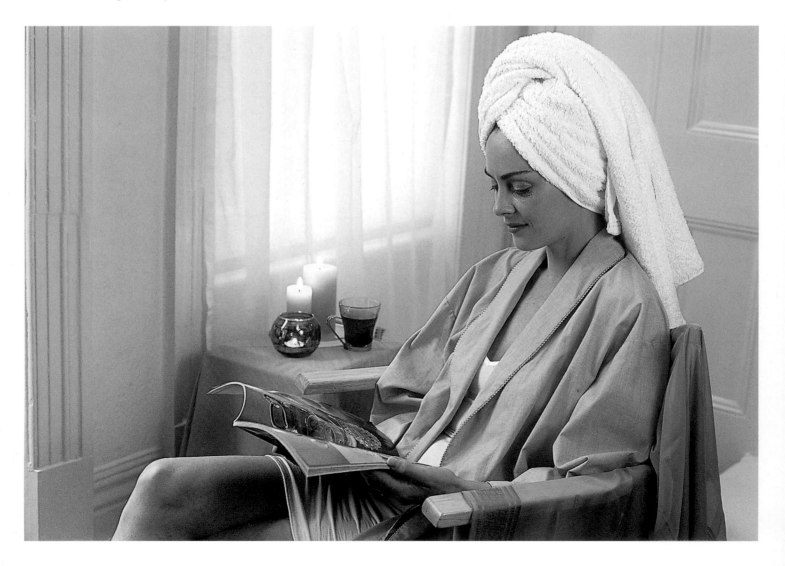

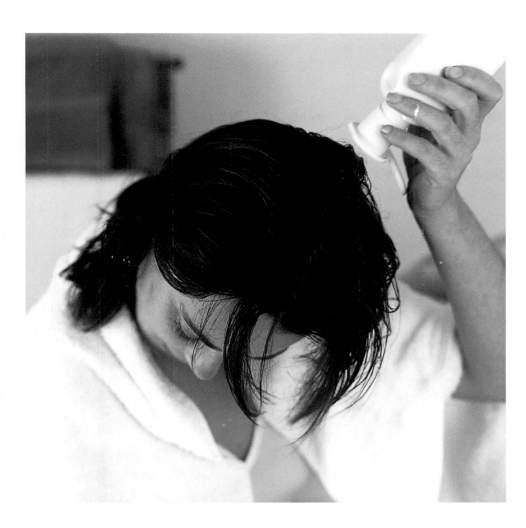

⊲ **When removing oils, always apply liberal quantities of shampoo directly onto the hair itself and work it repeatedly into the hair shafts and scalp before rinsing.**

in, shampoo again for a third time, working it in as before. When this stage is finished you are ready for rinsing.

Using warm water (once again the temperature will help break down any residual oil), thoroughly rinse out the shampoo. For a final time, shampoo your hair again. Your hair should be a mass of lather and soapsuds by now, so you should only need to use a little shampoo for this final wash. Rinse out as usual. Your hair is now ready for your usual drying and styling.

aftercare

To maintain the good you've just done to your hair, follow some of the advice suggested in the section on hair care. Particularly, try to leave your hair to dry naturally if you have the time. If you only have a little time to spare, and need to use a hairdryer, remove any excess water from the hair by towel-drying it first. This reduces the drying effects of a hairdryer.

▽ **Your hair should be free of oil and full of foamy suds by the end of the oil-removing session. It should be in tip-top condition.**

If you plan to leave the oils on overnight, then you may find it more comfortable to have the hair loose and use old towels or sheets to protect the bedding.

removing oils

When it comes to removing the oil from your hair, it is vital to use lots of shampoo at the start.

Do not wet your hair, but put the shampoo on first. If you put water on your hair it will interfere with the break down of the oil molecules and will make the oil harder to remove – it's the same principle as using oil paint and then trying to clean your brush with water. On the other hand, shampoo without water emulsifies with the oil, making it easier to rinse out later. You will probably need to use a lot of shampoo, but don't be alarmed at the amount you are using as it will take a lot to get the oil out of the hair. It is unlikely at this stage that you'll notice any lather. Once you have thoroughly shampooed your whole head, begin the whole process again as if you were starting from scratch.

Still without water, shampoo over your whole head and hair, working it well into the hair fibres. If you have long hair, take a handful and rub it between your hands as if you were scrubbing. At this point, it is likely that you will begin to see some lather. This is a good sign and indicates that you are well on the way to being able to wash out the oil successfully. Work your way round the whole head, rubbing your hair between your hands. When this is all worked

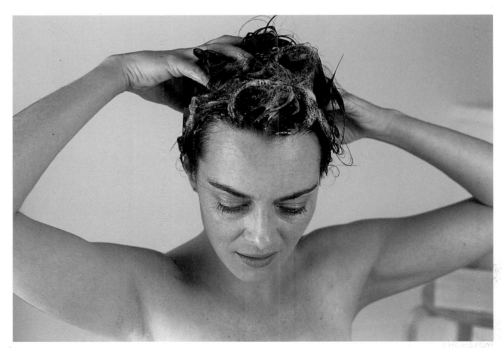

oil massage with a partner

Sometimes you and your massage partner may decide to opt for using oils when giving a head massage. Sharing an oil massage can be an enriching experience, depending on the need at the time and the oils used. It will add another dimension to the routines described elsewhere in the book. Oils also make it easier to extend a treatment to take in a general back and upper-body massage.

From a wide range of oils to choose from, you can make up your own concoctions to suit the particular situation – to enhance moods, relieve physical conditions or to facilitate emotional and physical healing. Take some time to assess your partner's particular need, and together choose the oils that seem most appropriate.

You can use a carrier oil on its own or you can add essential oils to the base oil for a broader effect. Several useful oil blends are suggested below. If you need more information on oils generally, see earlier pages in this chapter.

a sensual experience

A massage that involves any kind of oil feels very different from one without, as the increased lubrication is smoother and feels more sensual. The addition of aromas to the oils can make the massage even more luxurious, shifting the emphasis from mainly therapeutic to something more special.

Using oils also enables you to extend a head massage to include an upper-body massage and so share a more relaxing and intimate experience with your partner. You can follow all the steps in the lying-down routine, but the oils will give the massage a very different character.

Warm your hands before applying oil, and use wide stroking movements to spread the oil evenly over the surface of your partner's skin. Apply more oil to the skin

▽ As you apply nourishing oil to your massage partner's body allow your hands to mould over the contours in a smooth gliding way, with long stroking movements.

essential oil blends
Outlined here are a range of useful essential oil combinations that are appropriate for a range of needs and conditions. Use 2 drops essential oil for every 10ml (2 tsp) carrier oil. Sweet almond is one of the best multi-purpose carrier oils you can use.
general aches and pains: lavender and rosemary
stress: sandalwood, lavender and geranium
mild depression: geranium and lavender
pampering and nourishment: sandalwood or geranium, mixed with coconut base oil because of its softening qualities
spiritual transformation: include frankincense, as this helps to break links with the past and facilitates moving forwards.

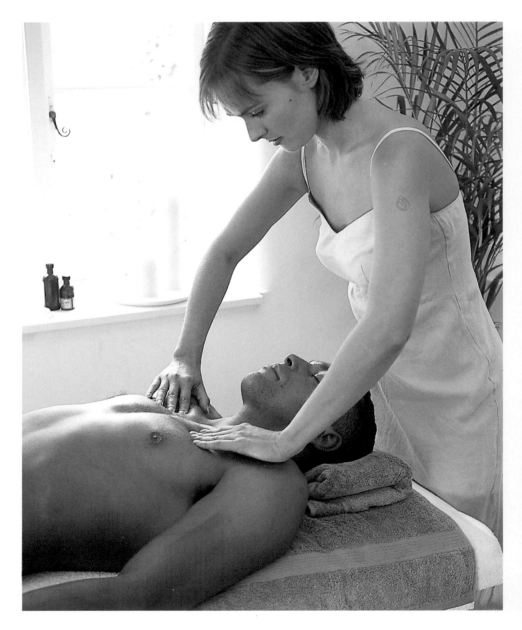

as you need to, but remember to always keep your other hand on your partner's body in order to keep the flow and a sense of continuity. Stroking, holding, circling and smoothing strokes can all be used effectively anywhere on the body when you are using oils.

Allow the nature of the oil as a medium to guide how you work. The oil on your hands will enable them to glide smoothly over your partner's skin. It will also make it easier for them to mould over the shape of the body and to follow its natural undulations. The strokes you use will be more gliding, stroking, smoothing and caressing in nature. You should also let yourself work at a slower pace than you normally would and take pleasure in the sensual nature of the oil itself.

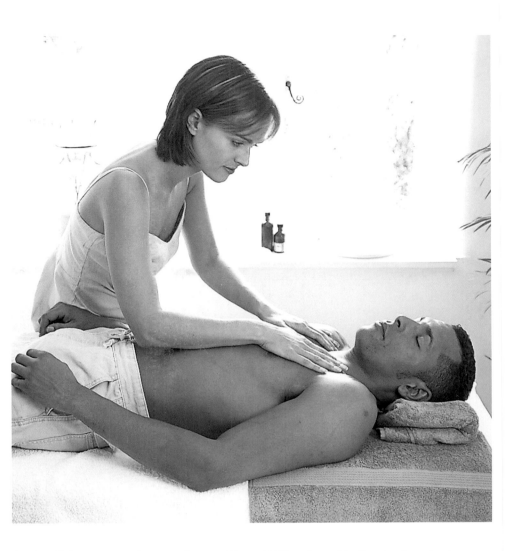

▽ Allow your hands to glide over the shoulders and back of the neck, easing out tension. Avoid working on the spine itself.

△ Using oils in a massage slows you down and if done regularly can be part of a real quality time with your partner as you connect on other levels.

▽ When done with oils, a tension-releasing shoulder massage can become a luxurious experience that is a pleasure to give and receive.

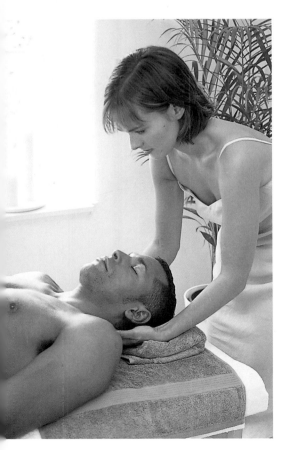

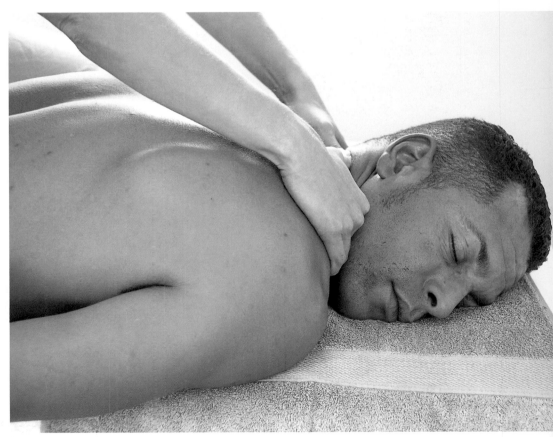

self-massage with oil

You may not think so at first, but giving yourself a head massage with oil can be as nourishing as receiving it from someone else. It is definitely worth trying, for it is very rewarding and is something that can easily be incorporated into your normal pampering and body-care routine. As oils have such a therapeutic effect, it would also be an ideal opportunity to extend the massage to other parts of the body, rubbing and smoothing oil on other areas, such as your arms, legs and feet as well as your face and neck. Always work up towards the heart when massaging other body parts.

getting started

Preparing the space for yourself is as important as if you were preparing it for someone else. Giving positive attention to creating the right atmosphere sends a strong message to your subconscious mind that you are worth it. This is a good opportunity to play self-healing or affirmation tapes, while relaxing background music will give you something to focus on if you feel bored. In Western culture we are not used to self-massage and reactions such as futility, doubt

▽ **Make sure that you have everything ready before you apply oils to your hands, as working with oils can be messy.**

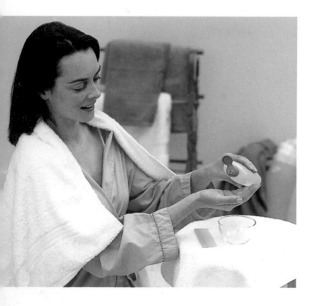

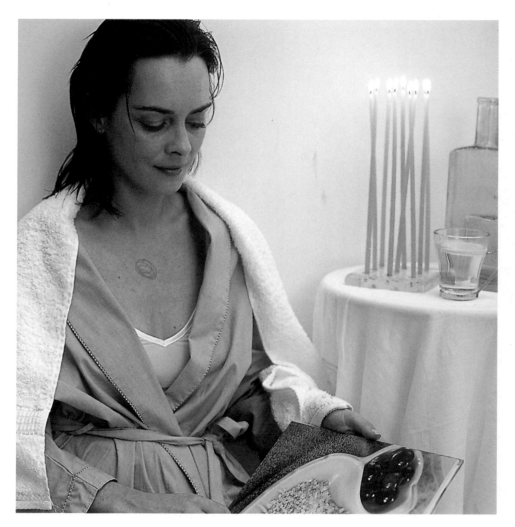

and dissatisfaction are common to begin with. Wear something loose and comfortable and that won't matter if it gets marked. Prepare everything else you may need for your pampering session. This will include a few towels to wrap yourself or your hair in, plenty of tissues, some water or herb tea and maybe some reading material and beauty preparations. You also need to have all the oils ready to hand plus a suitable mixing bowl and comb.

Warm up a little oil in the palm of your hand and apply it to the top of your head. Loosely ruffle your hair and work it in. Then apply some oil to the sides of your head and work this in. If you have long hair, you may need to lift it up and work outwards from the roots to the tips. Apply more oil, working from the front to the back of the

△ **Allowing time for the oils to sink in provides an opportunity to spend some quality time on yourself for self-nourishment and to rebalance. Use it to do something you really enjoy.**

head. Using the pads of your fingers, go on to make circular strokes across your scalp with medium pressure. Work methodically from the front to the back, covering the whole head. You should feel your scalp move underneath your fingers. When you have finished, cover your head and leave the oils to sink into your hair and scalp to do their work. This can be anything from 20 minutes to 24 hours. Using a warm towel around your head accelerates the penetration of the oils into the hair and scalp. Wrap it around your head "turban style" and use the time to catch up with yourself and relax.

▷ For a truly nourishing experience, use oils to help you massage away tensions and knots and to help create a greater sense of ease within your own body.

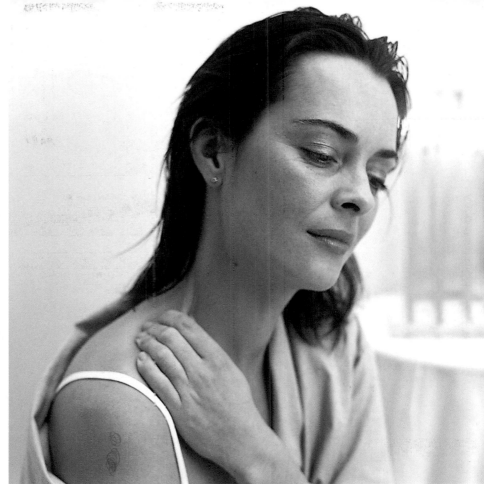

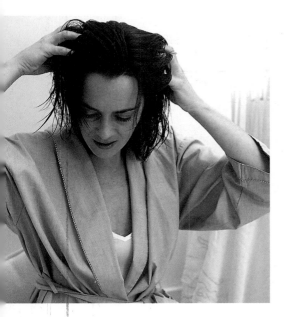

△ Release tension in the head and discharge mental stress and worries by working them out through massage and oils. Then you can wash them all away.

To continue working with oil you can follow the basic self-massage sequence outlined earlier in the book. However, because of its slippery nature there will be more "give" with oil and you will have less of a grip than with dry massage, so the experience will feel very different. With oils your strokes are likely to be smooth, gliding over the skin in a continuous movement.

After you have finished with your hair you may want to use up any remaining oil on your face and neck. Place your hands on your face and gently smooth the oil into the skin with small circular strokes, being particularly careful around the eyes. Move to your neck and glide your hands up and out to the sides. You can leave the oil to soak in or wipe it off with a tissue.

Remember that when giving self-massage you are both the giver and the receiver. As the giver you are your own therapist, so be sympathetic and understanding to how you feel inside. As you massage you could inwardly thank the different parts of your body for serving you

so well each day. You may also notice how your thoughts stray away or become negative, worrying or busy. When this happens, bring your attention back to the self-massage. As the receiver, you have the opportunity for self-empowerment and healing. If it hurts, you can instantly lighten the depth of your touch. Alternatively you can apply pressure for much longer than is conventional if it feels good to you. You also know exactly where it hurts and can find the precise location of any knotty and painful spots.

As you massage, make sure that your strokes give you pleasure, adjusting the pace so that it is faster, slower, deeper, or more loving. Be responsive to your own needs and be flexible in your approach. A basic guideline is to recognize that the body has a wisdom of its own and that if something feels good, it is likely to be doing you good.

▽ Relieve tension in your face with an oil facial that will leave you feeling good and your skin soft, smooth and glowing.

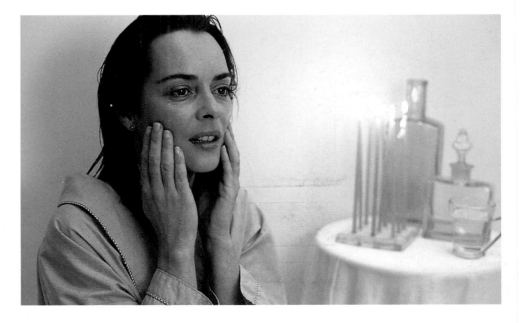

Natural hair care

The colour, thickness, texture and pattern of our hair are determined by our genetic make-up and are out of our control. What we do with what nature has given us however is up to us. Although commercial hair-care products may work to some extent, overall a more holistic approach is needed if we are to achieve the lustrous hair that most of us long for. Natural hair care involves looking after our general wellbeing and diet as well as finding practical ways to take care of our hair.

healthy living

The state of our hair is a good barometer of our general state of health. When we are ill or stressed our hair looks lank and lifeless. When we feel good we have a spring in our step and our hair has a bounce and shine. Strong hair growth is related to general vitality, sexual energy, balanced hormonal activity and having enough sleep and exposure to sunlight. It is also related to what we eat.

▽ Groom wet or oiled hair with a wide-toothed comb as this helps to prevent damage to the hair. It also allows it to dry naturally, so long as conditions make this possible.

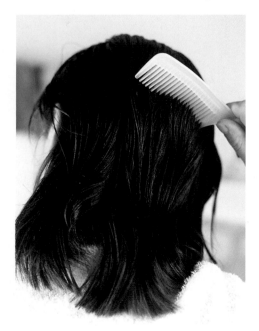

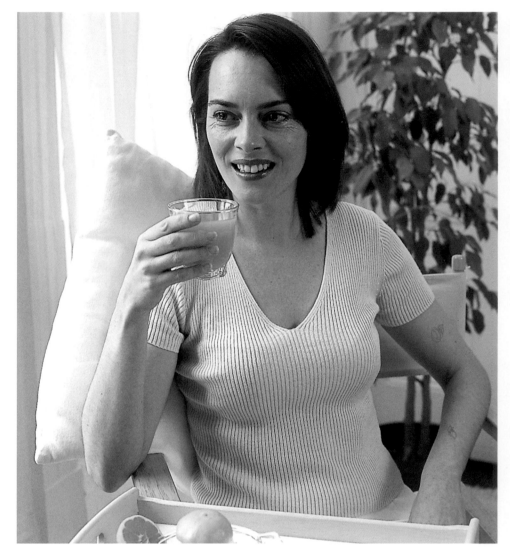

Maintaining a balanced diet is essential for building and maintaining healthy hair. This means eating plenty of whole grains, fresh vegetables and fruit. Seeds, nuts, olives and fish should be included in the diet and meat and dairy products in moderation. If you are making adjustments to your eating habits, don't be impatient for quick results; it takes three to four months for what we are eating to be reflected in the condition of our hair.

hair washing

In some cultures people do not shampoo their hair but have other treatments such as oiling or just washing with water. This idea may sound strange at first, but in fact when

△ Eat a wholesome diet that includes plenty of vegetables and fruit to provide the necessary nutrients for maintaining a vibrant and sensuous look to your hair.

left alone the hair reaches a point of homeostasis where it is protected by its natural oils and so there is no need for soap.

In our society the trend towards frequent hair washing is actually damaging to the hair. It strips it of all its natural oils and also dries out the scalp. This then stimulates the sebaceous glands to produce more oil to compensate, which then leads to greasy hair and more hair washing, and a vicious circle is created. To break the pattern, try to cut down how often you shampoo your hair

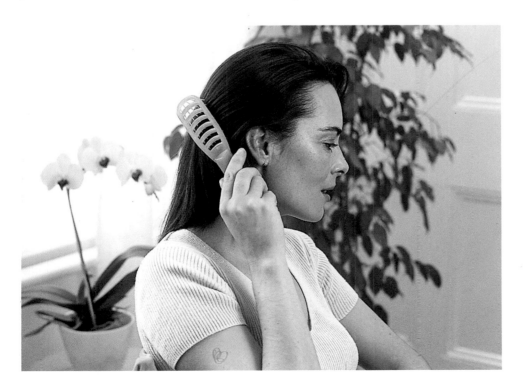

and get into the habit of using less shampoo, lathering up only once instead of twice.

Hair is most vulnerable to damage when it is wet, so it needs to be treated carefully. Use a wide-toothed comb and always start from the ends of the hair to avoid stretching the hair shaft. This is a good principle to apply even when the hair is dry.

hair drying

Ideally hair is best left to dry naturally as hairdryers have a damaging and drying-out effect on the hair. If you do use a hairdryer, try using it less often. A high-voltage dryer will reduce the time your hair is exposed to the intense heat. Towel-dry your hair first and then hold the dryer at least 15cm (6in) away from your head. If you use heated styling devices, such as rollers, irons or tongs, try to use them as infrequently and for as short a time as possible.

To keep your hair at its best, you need to protect it from the drying effects of the sea,

▽ Brushing your hair, rather than just combing it through, helps disperse the oils your head produces so that the whole of the hair benefits.

sun and the swimming pool. Before swimming, take a shower and get your hair thoroughly wet, as this will help it to absorb less salt or chlorine. You can protect your hair from the drying effects of the sun and wind by wearing a hat.

hair dyes

Research suggests that there may be some risks associated with using chemical dyes on the hair, as the dyes are absorbed into the bloodstream through the scalp and could be toxic to the body. There are many plant- or vegetable-based dyes available that do not pose this risk.

△ Using henna and natural hair dyes introduces colour but minimizes the potential health risks associated with some commercial chemicals.

common hair problems
The following hair problems are all helped by head massage.

greasy hair
Head massage will stimulate the sebaceous glands to work properly and help prevent the hair follicles from clogging up with sebum. Jojoba oil helps to regulate over-productive sebaceous glands. For hair washing, use mild shampoos and avoid washing too often.

dry hair
Head massage combined with regular hot-oil treatments is ideal for conditioning and moisturizing dry hair. Ideally you should leave the oil in overnight. Avoid hair products that contain isopropyl or ethyl alcohol, which dry the hair.

hair loss
Head massage will have a stimulating effect, speeding up the delivery of nutrients to the roots and hair shaft and encouraging new hair growth.

Natural face refreshers

Our facial muscles are in constant use. They respond to our inner thoughts and feelings, as well as stress and tension from the outside. Without release, these tensions build up over time and contribute to the formation of facial lines and wrinkles, making us look much older than our years. A furrowed brow, a mouth that is slightly pulled down at the corners, eyes that have a hard look and pale, dry or tired-looking skin are all signs of stress and facial tension. Fortunately there are many ways to counteract some of these effects without recourse to cosmetic surgery or expensive beauty preparations. These methods include facial massage, stretching exercises and other natural quick-fix treatments.

instant effects

The astonishing thing about facial massage is that its effects are immediate and tangible. The combination of working with oils, massage and pressure points can result in an immediate restoration of natural beauty and vitality, eliminating lines and wrinkles caused by stressed muscles; improving skin colour and tone, restoring shine and sparkle to dull, tired eyes. Done regularly, it can also help to delay signs of ageing by boosting facial muscle tone and improving the general appearance of the skin through more efficient circulation, skin nutrition and the elimination of toxins. Because the surface of the face has so many nerve receptors, facial massage is also very effective at sending relaxing signals to the brain, which in turn calms and relaxes the mind and helps the body to relax even more.

quick massage routine

Before you begin a facial massage you need to release the muscles of the scalp first. This is because any tightness in the scalp has a pulling effect on the facial muscles, registering as a tight or pinched look. To do this follow the strokes shown in Self Massage, the Head, then proceed with this quick facial massage.

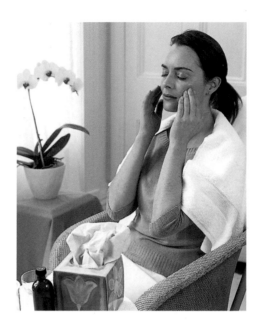

△ **1** Rest your palms against the sides of your face with your fingertips resting on your cheekbones. Using light pressure, slide your fingertips up either side of the nose and through the forehead. Continue across your forehead and down the sides of your face to finish in the middle of the jawbone. Repeat this circuit three times.

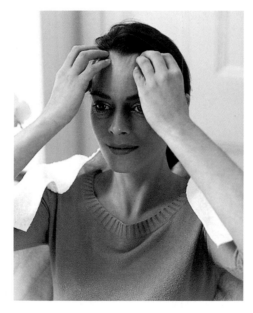

△ **2** Put your fingertips by the frown line in the centre of your eyebrows. With medium pressure, slide these fingers upwards and outwards towards the temples, smoothing out any tension lines as you go. Repeat three times.

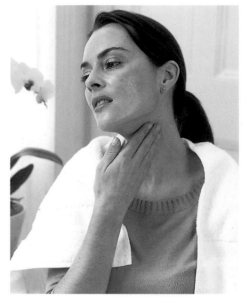

△ **3** Add a little more oil to your hands, then smooth it from your collarbone up your neck using the flat part of your fingers. Work across from the front to the back of your neck, extending the stroke to use the flats of your hands. Remember to only use pressure when your hands move in an upward direction, as you don't want to pull the skin down. To release the muscles at the neck, make large spiralling circles up the sides of the neck, finishing at the hairline at the base of the skull.

using facial oils

Although you can massage the face dry, using a little oil is nourishing for the skin and helps your fingers to glide more smoothly. It also makes it more of a pampering experience. There is a variety of suitable oils, depending on your skin type and personal preference. Rose facial oil is particularly luxurious, while wheat-germ oil is very rich in vitamin E, which is nourishing and lubricating for the skin. Alternatively almond, apricot and/or jojoba oil are all good choices, as they are easily absorbed by the skin.

▷ Keeping the skin hydrated is essential. In addition to drinking water you can freshen up with a water-based spritzer.

facial stretches

To finish your natural facelift treatment, a few facial stretches will tone and strengthen the muscles and help to firm up your face. They will also help you to release any remaining facial tension and leave you looking refreshed and rejuvenated.

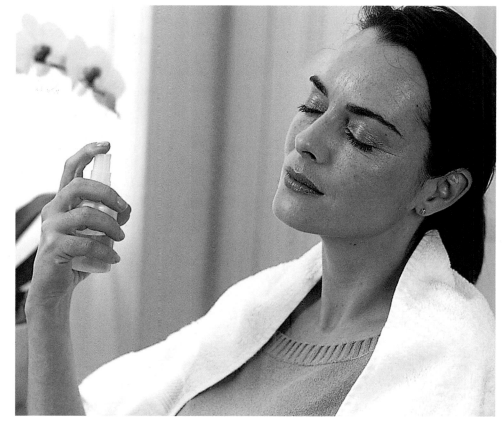

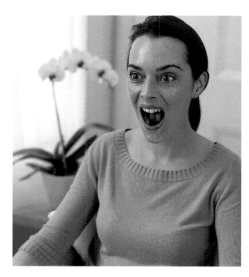

△ **1** To give your face a good stretch, open your mouth wide, raise your eyebrows and widen your eyes at the same time. Hold for 5 seconds and then relax and let go. Repeat twice more.

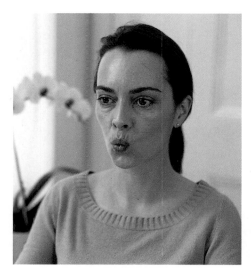

△ **2** Take a deep breath in, and on the out breath suck both your cheeks in at the same time. Hold for 5 seconds and as you hold, try sucking your cheeks in a little further, particularly around the jaw socket area. Release and repeat twice more.

facial refreshers

Water is essential to fresh-looking skin, and as well as various stretches, massage routines and exercises it is also important to keep your skin hydrated. Being adequately hydrated keeps the body's internal organs working efficiently and helps maintain the skin's elasticity. It is recommended that we drink a minimum of 2 litres (3½ pints) a day. To counter the drying effects of the weather, heating and air conditioning, our skin may also need additional support. You can give your skin a quick boost by spraying water on to your face with a mist sprayer, or by splashing tap water on to it.

To refresh and rejuvenate puffy eyes, place a slice of cucumber over each eye and lie back with your eyes closed. Relax and rest for a few minutes as the cucumber juice seeps into your skin. The juice from cucumbers contains valuable properties, which sooth and refresh tired eyes.

▽ **Eyes are often the first thing to register and reveal our state of being. Soothing cucumber will help relieve tension and tiredness.**

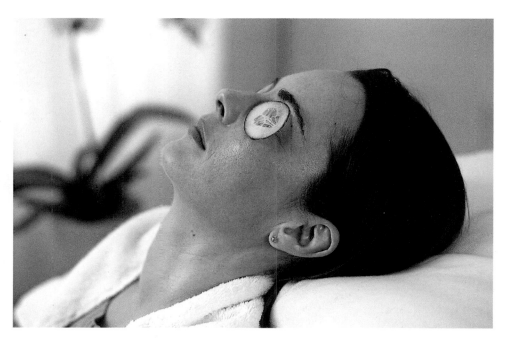

Bibliography

Acknowledgements

Atkinson, Mary *The Art of Indian Head Massage* (Carlton Books Ltd 2000)

Ayres, Professor Jon *Asthma* (Dorling Kindersley Ltd 1999)

Bentley, Eilean *Step by Step Head Massage* (Cygnus Books 2000)

Crane, Beryl *Reflexology the Definitive Practioner's Manual* (Element Books 1997)

Davis, Patricia *Aromatherapy A–Z* (C W Daniel Company Ltd 1995)

Field, T; Henteleff, T; Hernandez-Reif, M; Kuhn, C; Martinez, E; Mavunda, K; and Schanberg, S. "Children with Asthma have Improved Pulmonary Functions after Massage Therapy" (*Journal of Pediatrics* 1997)

Fox, Su and Pritchard, Darien *Anatomy, Physiology and Pathology for the Massage Therapist* (Corpus Publishing 2001)

Fulton, Susan "An Introduction to Head Massage" (Video, IMC Vision 2001)

Gach Reed, Michael *Accupressure* (Piatkus Ltd 1992)

Maxwell Hudson, Clare *Massage* (Dorling Kindersley Ltd 2001)

McGuinness, Helen *Head Massage* (Hodder and Stoughton 2000)

Mehta, Narendra *Indian Head Massage* (Thorsons – an imprint of HarpersCollins Publishers 1999)

Schneider, Meir and Larkin, Maureen with Schneider, Dror *The Handbook of Self Healing* (Penguin Group 1994)

Schulman, K R and Jones, G E "The Effectiveness of Massage Intervention on Reducing Anxiety in the Workplace" (*Journal of Applied Behavioural Science* 1996)

Vyas, Bharti with Haggard, Claire *Beauty Wisdom* (Thorsons – an imprint of HarpersCollins Publishers 1997)

Widdowson, Rosalind *Head Massage* (Octopus Publishing Group Ltd 2000)

Wischik, Lucian "A Whirlwind Tour through the Entire History of Massage" (www.wischik.com/lu/massage)

Worth, Jennifer "One Hundred Years of Treating Asthma" (*Positive Health*, April 2002)

Worwood, Valerie Ann *The Fragrant Pharmacy* (Macmillan London Ltd 1990 Bantam edition 1991)

I am grateful to my children Sam, Joe and Ben for inspiring me and for their generosity in putting up with me while writing this book. I have valued Sam's realism, Joe's clarity and patient computer support, and Ben's enthusiasm.

Thanks also to therapists Karine Buchart, Jocelyn Ford Beazley, Susie Berkeley, Liz, Sulia Rose, Ibrahim Lingwood, Susan Harwood and Amanda Lindsey, for their professional input, and to Joanne of Anness Publishing for her incisive clarity and direction.

I acknowledge Amanda Relph for her encouragement and the use of her beautiful home for photo shoots. Thank you to my parents and friends, especially Diane, for encouragement and to all the other helpers, seen and unseen.

Picture acknowledgements
Thanks to the following agencies for permission to use their images:
The Bridgeman Art Library; p10 bottom left, p11, p12 bottom left.
Corbis; p13 bottom, p15 top right & top left, p82 top.
Sylvia Cordaiy; p12 top right, p14 bottom left.

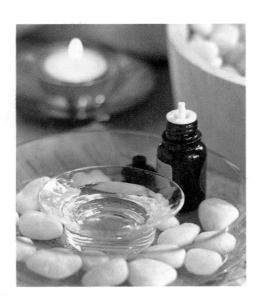

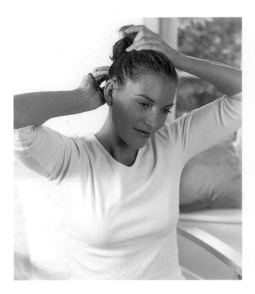

Index

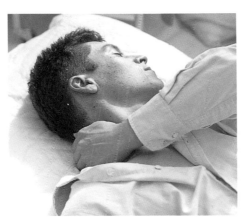

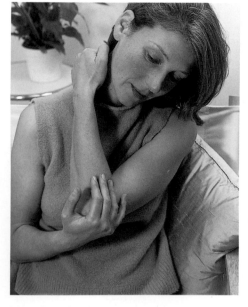
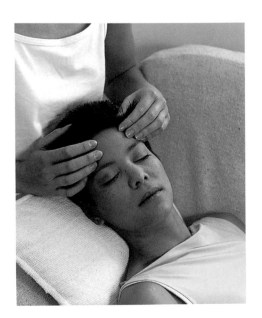

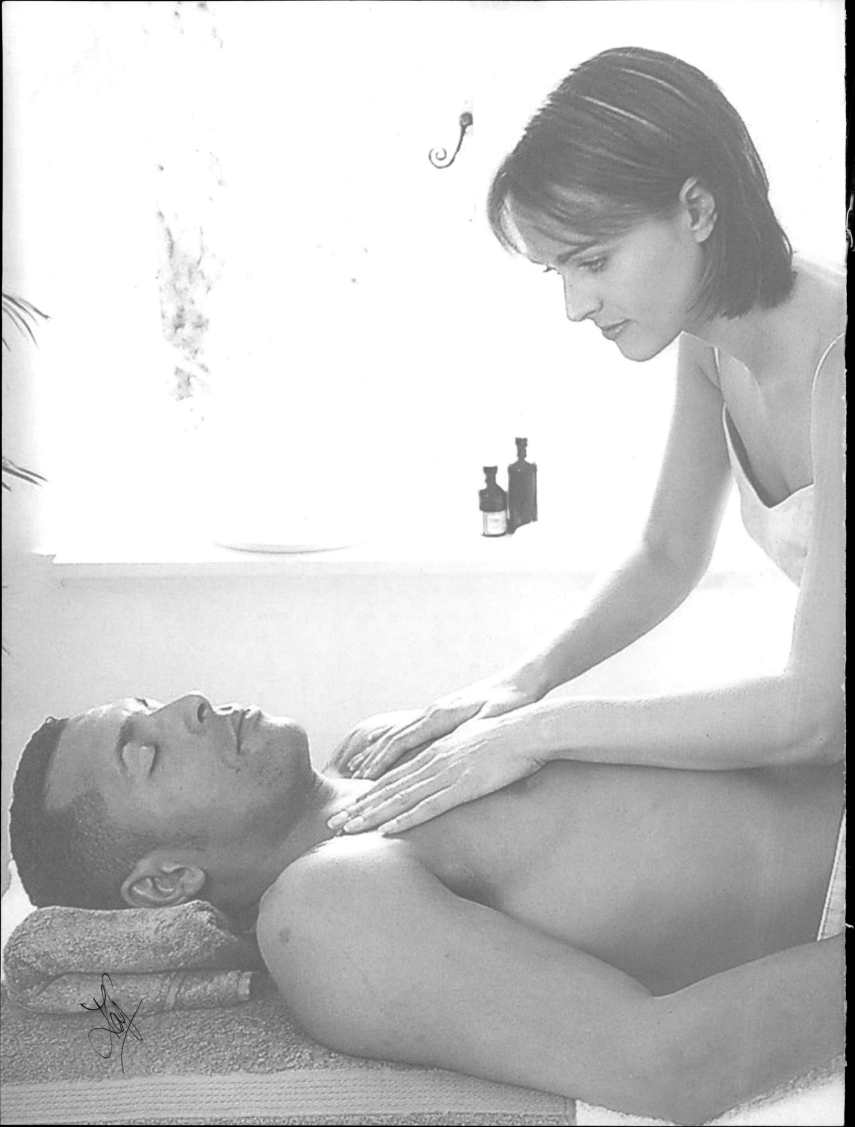

Index

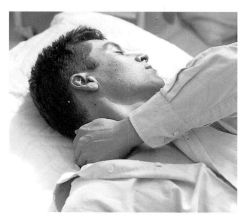

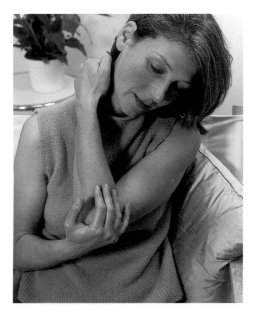

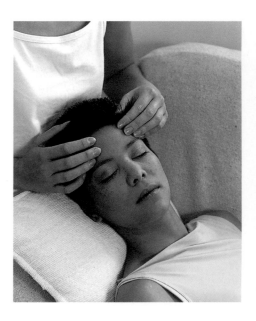

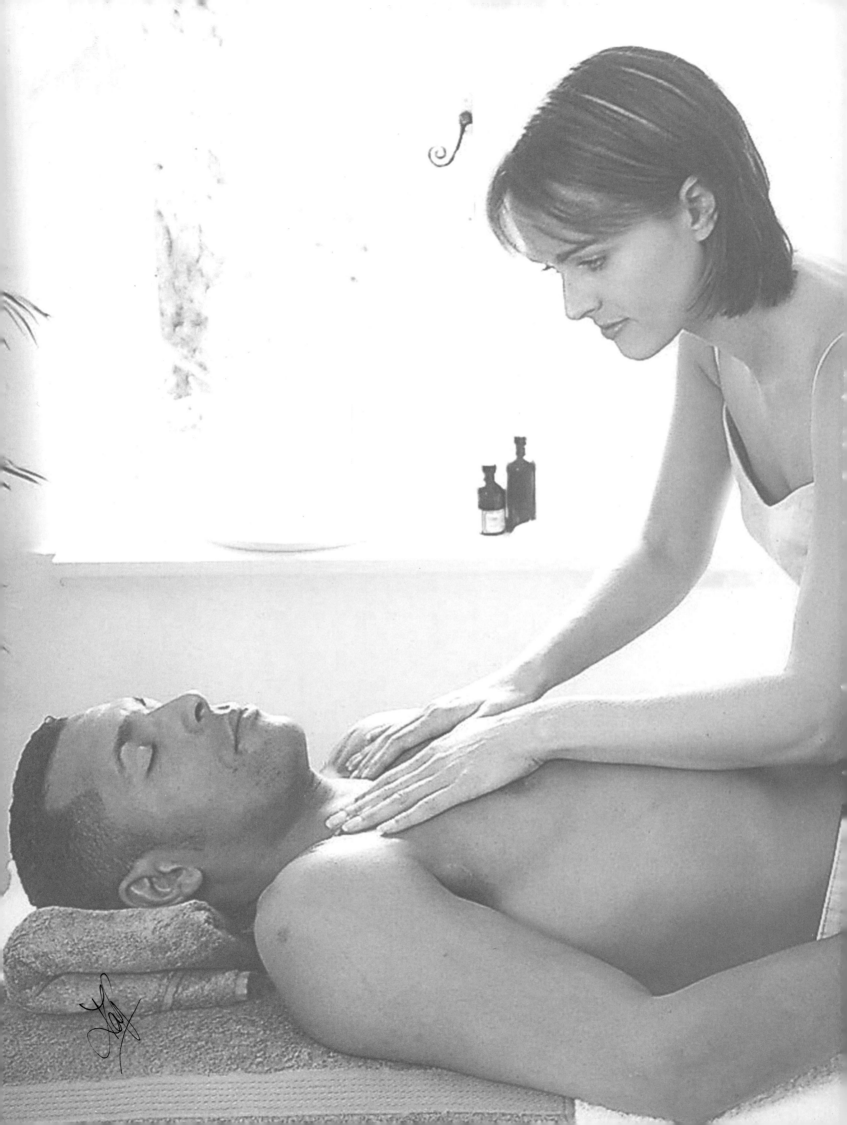